Clinical Talk

Cardiology to Impress

The Ultimate Guide for Students and Junior Doctors

CLINICAL TALK

Series Editors: Andrew Goldberg *(University College London and the Royal National Orthopaedic Hospital NHS Trust, Stanmore, UK)*
Gerard Stansby *(University of Newcastle and Freeman Hospital, Newcastle Hospitals NHS Trust, UK)*

Published:

Surgery: Problems and Solutions
Revision Questions in Undergraduate Surgery
edited by Andrew Goldberg (University College London and the Royal National Orthopaedic Hospital NHS Trust, Stanmore, UK) and Gerard Stansby (University of Newcastle and Freeman Hospital, Newcastle Hospitals NHS Trust, UK)

Forthcoming:

Core Clinical Medicine
by Gordon W Stewart (University College London, UK)

CLINICAL TALK

Cardiology to Impress

The Ultimate Guide for Students and Junior Doctors

Kathie Wong | Edith Ubogagu | Darrel Francis

Imperial College London, UK

Series Editors

Andrew Goldberg

University College London and the

Royal National Orthopaedic Hospital NHS Trust, Stanmore, UK

Gerard Stansby

University of Newcastle and Freeman Hospital,

Newcastle Hospitals NHS Trust, UK

ICP

Imperial College Press

Published by

Imperial College Press
57 Shelton Street
Covent Garden
London WC2H 9HE

Distributed by

World Scientific Publishing Co. Pte. Ltd.
5 Toh Tuck Link, Singapore 596224
USA office: 27 Warren Street, Suite 401-402, Hackensack, NJ 07601
UK office: 57 Shelton Street, Covent Garden, London WC2H 9HE

British Library Cataloguing-in-Publication Data
A catalogue record for this book is available from the British Library.

Clinical Talk
CARDIOLOGY TO IMPRESS
The Ultimate Guide for Students and Junior Doctors

ISBN-13 978-1-84816-538-0 (pbk)
ISBN-10 1-84816-538-2 (pbk)

Typeset by Stallion Press
Email: enquiries@stallionpress.com

Printed in Singapore by Mainland Press Pte Ltd

Dedications

Edith: Gratitude first and foremost to God! Philippians 4:13. I am indebted to my family and friends for all their support especially my mother, and finally to my co-authors, without whom this would not have been possible.

Kathie: To my mother for giving me her strength and creativity. To my family and friends for all their support. Special thanks to Imperial College Press for giving us this opportunity.

Contributors: Dr. Ashoke Roy and Dr. Christina Papadopoulos

Preface

The ultimate firm guide for medical students preparing them for the clinical experience. This book is written by newly qualified doctors who are familiar with the pitfalls of clinical attachments and who understand the fears and apprehensions when students are thrown into the hospital setting. This pocket-size handbook specifically outlines what medical students are to expect, and what is expected of them when sitting in clinics and theatres. It addresses how not to look like a fool in front of senior doctors and provides hints and tips on how to answer questions on ward rounds. It is not designed to replace medical textbooks but is a down-to-earth relay of experience from a student perspective, bridging the gap between textbook knowledge and clinical practice.

This guidebook has been written in collaboration with top teaching consultants who are familiar with the gaps of knowledge of the average medical student. It does not aim to cover the minutia of cardiovascular medicine, rather it aims to deal with subjects students struggle to understand, subjects that are ill-defined in mainstream textbooks. It is written in an informal, story-telling style, avoiding unnecessary jargon.

This is the hands-on tool providing up-to-date information in one of the most rapidly evolving fields in medicine. Coronary heart disease is the number one killer in the western world. Therefore, a comprehensive knowledge in this field is essential for the student and applicable regardless of whichever speciality they later embark on. This instrument is specifically designed to fit into your handbag thereby making it the ideal companion on long journeys to and from attachments. By the end of it, students should be confident, competent in their skills, with better insight into evidence-based practice. We hope to stimulate an interest in cardiology and that its launch will be a debut to a potential series of guidebooks for medical students in other clinical specialities.

Kathie and Edith

Contents

List of Abbreviations

4S	— Scandinavian Simvastatin Survival Study
AF	— atrial fibrillation
ALLHAT	— Antihypertensive and Lipid-Lowering Treatment to Prevent Heart Attack Trial
ALS	— adult life support
APSIS	— angina prognosis study in Stockholm
AR	— aortic regurgitation
ARVC	— arrhythmogenic right ventricular cardiomyopathy
AS	— aortic stenosis
ASCOT	— Anglo-Scandinavian Cardiac Outcomes Trial
ASD	— atrial septal defect
ASH	— asymmetrical septal hypertrophy
AVID	— Antiarrhythmics Versus Implantable Defibrillators
AVNRT	— atrioventricular nodal re-entry tachycardia
BCT	— broad complex tachycardia
B(I)D	— 'bis in die' (twice a day)
BNF	— British National Formulary
CABG	— coronary artery bypass graft
CARE	— Cholesterol and Recurrent Events trial
CASH	— Cardiac Arrest Study Hamburg
CCB	— calcium channel blocker
CHD	— coronary heart disease
CIBIS II	— Cardiac Insufficiency Bisoprolol Study II
CID	— Canadian Implantable Defibrillator Study

CONSENSUS — Cooperative North Scandinavian Enalapril Survival Study
CREST — calcinosis, Raynaud's syndrome, oesophageal dysmotility, scleroderma, telangectasia
CRT — cardiac resynchronisation therapy
CRT-D — cardiac resynchronisation therapy with a defibrillator
CRT-P — cardiac resynchronisation therapy with a pacemaker
CXR — chest X-ray
CT — computerised tomography
DBP — diastolic blood pressure
DCCV — direct current cardioversion
DCM — dilated cardiomyopathy
ECG — electrocardiogram
EF — ejection fraction
ELITE — Evaluation of Losartan in The Elderly Study
ESM — ejection systolic murmur
FBC — full blood count
GP — general practitioner
HAPPHY — Heart Attack Primary Prevention in Hypertension trial
H(O)CM — hypertrophic (obstructive) cardiomyopathy
HOPE — Heart Outcomes Prevention Evaluation Study
ICD — implantable cardiac defibrillator
INVEST — International Verapamil SR/Tradolapril study
ISIS 4 — Fourth International Study of Infarct Survival
IV — intravenous
JVP — jugular venous pressure
LBBB — left bundle branch block
LVH — left ventricular hypertrophy
MADIT — multicenter automatic defibrillator implantation trial
MEN — multiple endocrine neoplasia
MERIT — Metoprolol CR/XL Randomised Intervention Trial

MI	— myocardial infarction
MR	— mitral regurgitation
MRI	— magnetic resonance imaging
MS	— mitral stenosis
MUGA	— multi gated acquisition scan
MUSTT	— Multicenter Unsustained Tachycardia Trial
NICE	— National Institute of health and Clinical Excellence
NSTEMI	— Non-ST-Elevation Myocardial Infarction
OD	— 'omni die' (once a day)
PCI	— percutaneous coronary intervention
PDA	— patent ductus arteriosus
PE	— pulmonary embolism
PLAATO	— percutaneous left atrial appendage transcatheter occlusion
PND	— paroxysmal nocturnal dyspnoea
PO	— per os (orally)
PRN	— 'pro re nata' as needed
RALES	— Randomised Aldactone Evaluation Study
RBBB	— right bundle branch block
RCM	— restrictive cardiomyopathy
RCT	— randomised controlled trial
RVH	— right ventricular hypertrophy
SAM	— systolic anterior motion of the mitral valve
SBP	— systolic blood pressure
SLE	— systemic lupus erythematosus
STEMI	— ST-Elevation Myocardial Infarction
SVT	— supraventricular tachycardia
TIA	— transient ischaemic attack
TIBET	— The Total Ischaemic Burden European Trial
TOE	— transoesophageal echocardiogram
TPA	— tissue plasminogen activator
UA	— unstable angina
U&E	— urea and electrolytes
VeHT	— Valsartan Heart Failure Trial
VF	— ventricular fibrillation

VT	— ventricular tachycardia
VTE	— venous thromboembolism
VSD	— ventral septal defect
WHO	— World health organisation
WPW	— Wolff-Parkinson-White syndrome

Chapter 1

Clerking Patients

Clerking patients may seem a daunting task initially, but it is an important skill to master. A well performed history and examination allows you to not only reach an appropriate differential diagnosis, and thus request relevant investigations, but also to develop an effective doctor–patient relationship. This chapter will ensure that you structure your history taking, and will point out the important questions to ask. It will help you to focus on understanding symptomatology, common abnormal examination findings and your presentation technique.

1.1 History Taking

It is vital to have a structure, at least in your head, on which to base your history as the patient rarely gives you the information needed in an orderly fashion.

The key cardiac symptoms are:

- Chest pain
- Dyspnoea
- Palpitations
- Oedema
- Syncope

1.1.1 *Five simple steps to taking a cardiac history*

Step 1: Ask about the presenting complaint:

Also make sure you cover the following, which are the main cardiac symptoms:

- chest pain
- dyspnoea/shortness of breath

- palpitations
- syncope
- oedema.

Bear in mind that none of the above symptoms are cardiac *specific*; they can be caused by non-cardiac pathology, and therefore thoughtful *directed* questioning of each symptom can help determine its cause. If a patient presents with any one of these symptoms, do not forget to enquire about the others. Try to keep in mind the causes of each symptom, as this will help direct your questioning.

Step 2: Always ask about the five major risk factors, namely:

- high blood pressure
- hypercholesterolaemia
- smoking
- diabetes

} *all modifiable*

- family history of cardiac disease — *non-modifiable.*

Step 3: Don't neglect the past medical history, including:

- heart disease and previous cardiac investigations or procedures including angioplasty/stent/bypass grafting
- history of stroke/transient ischaemic attack
- history of peripheral vascular disease
- asthma — as B-blockers and adenosine can cause bronchospasm
- rheumatic fever — predisposition to valve disease
- thyroid disease — can cause palpitations and exacerbate heart failure.

Step 4: A full drug history:

- remember that patients don't often list aspirin or inhalers spontaneously
- any drug allergies? *Be specific* — patients do not always understand this question. Did the patient have an anaphylactic reaction/rash/nausea/vomiting, or did they simply not benefit from taking the drug?

Step 5: Patient's social circumstances:

- occupation (for example, taxi drivers and airline pilots have strict occupational health regulations)
- implications post-myocardial infarction
- who lives at home with the patient?
- pre-morbid health — before this admission what was the patient's level of independence and activity? Gives an idea on what to aim for prior to discharge
- alcohol history — predisposition to hypertension, cardiomyopathy and atrial fibrillation.

1.2 Chest Pain

Chest pain is a simple shorthand that we use to describe a wide variety of experiences. You'll be surprised at how often you and the patient may not be referring to the same thing! For example, does the patient mean an ache, heartburn, or heaviness in the chest? Finding out the nature or characteristics of the pain can provide important clues as to whether or not the pain is cardiac in nature.

There are two critical features of *cardiac* chest pain:

1. **Location** of the pain may be typically symmetrical across the centre of the chest, potentially including both shoulders and arms, and may radiate up the neck to the jaw. It may be more dominant on the left side.
2. **Exertional relationship** — coronary pain will always get worse when the patient is physically active. Pain that occurs randomly at rest and during exercise with no exertional link is usually non-cardiac in origin. Pain that has a habitual pattern of only occurring at rest is very unlikely to be cardiac.

Ask about associated shortness of breath and autonomic symptoms such as nausea and sweatiness. Glyceryl trinitrate (GTN) will usually offer some symptom relief, whether the patient is experiencing angina or a myocardial infarction. However, if pain lasts for more than

20 minutes with or without relief by GTN, consideration of a myocardial infarction (MI) is warranted.

1.2.1 *The key features of cardiac chest pain*

- crushing pain/tightness over central chest
- +/– radiation to jaw/down the left arm
- +/– autonomic symptoms, for example, nausea, sweatiness

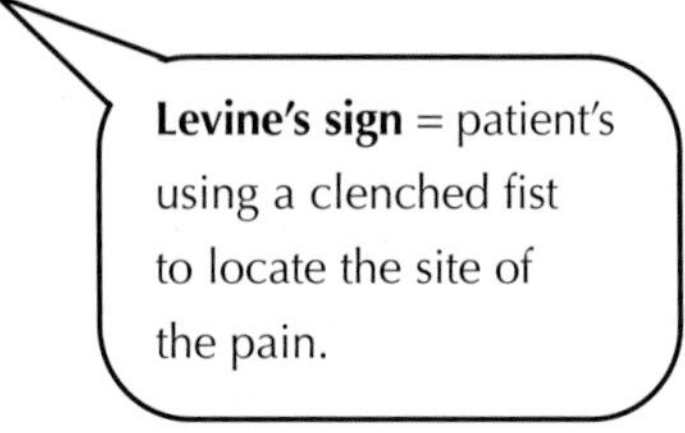

Other cardiac causes of chest pain include:

- *Aortic dissection* — this is a life-threatening condition where blood is tracking between the layers of the wall of the aorta. Left untreated, there is a high risk of rupture and death. This is characterised by a 'tearing' central chest pain radiating to the back between the scapulae. May be accompanied by haemodynamic compromise.
- *Pericarditis* — this is inflammation of the pericardium which causes chest pain worse on inspiration or lying flat.
- *Arrhythmias* — these can sometimes cause chest pain if the rate becomes really fast.

The main non-cardiac causes of chest pain that are often mistaken for angina can be divided into **respiratory, gastrointestinal** and **musculoskeletal** causes. For example, *sharp* chest pain is often referred to as *pleuritic* chest pain and is suggestive of a pleuritic/respiratory cause, such as an infection (for example, pneumonia), inflammation (for example, pleurisy), or infarction (for example, a Pulmonary Embolism [PE]). It is caused by inflamed contact between the lung and pleura.

Some important differentiating questions for pleuritic pain include:

- Is it worse on deep inspiration? On coughing? With movement?
- Is the pain sharp? Like a sharp knife? Note that some patients will use the word 'sharp' to mean 'severe' rather than to describe the type of pain.

Consider a **gastrointestinal cause** such as oesophagitis, oesophageal reflux or spasm if the chest pain is *burning* and is worse on lying flat or is related to meals. Pain that is relieved on sitting forward may suggest pancreatitis.

- Is the pain worse in any one position? Such as lying flat?
- Is the pain relieved by sitting forward?
- Is the pain worse before/after eating?

Don't forget musculoskeletal/cutaneous chest pain which is confined to the chest wall and may be tender on palpation, for example, Tietze's syndrome (costochondritis = inflammation of the costal cartilages), or herpes zoster (shingles), which can also give rise to a vesicular rash on the chest wall in a dermatomal distribution.

You can use the questions based on the well-known mnemonic SOCRATES below to guide your history taking.

S — Site: Where is the pain?
O — Onset: When did the pain first start?
C — Character: Describe the pain.
R — Radiation: Does the pain spread anywhere?
A — Associated symptoms: Any nausea, pallor, sweating or dizziness?
T — Timing and duration: How long does the pain last?
E — Exacerbating and relieving factors: This includes drug treatment, that is, GTN.
S — Severity: Score out of ten. (Ten being the worse pain the patient has ever experienced.)

Despite learning all of these well recognised patterns of chest pain, some patients may have *atypical* chest pain; that is, chest pain that doesn't follow the typical pattern of presentation for the disease. For example, a patient with a myocardial infarction may present with only left arm pain, or shortness of breath. They may even present with *pleuritic* sounding, *sharp* chest pain or heartburn. Pain that is very well localised or point-like, that is, a pain that the patient can point to with a fingertip, rarely turns out to be coronary in origin. Multifocal pain is also very unlikely to be cardiac in origin as coronary chest pain is characteristically stereotyped within any one single individual in the core location in which it affects, although as it becomes more severe it can radiate to more areas. Furthermore, some patients may not experience any chest pain at all, particularly those who are elderly, with diabetes, and/or following cardiac transplantation. It is thought that the weakening of the peripheral nerve function (through age, diabetes, or heart transplant surgery) prevents the information travelling to the brain in the way that typically causes pain.

Multifocal pain describes pain that occurs randomly at various points across the chest which may all present at the same time.

Radiation on the other hand, implies a more temporal relationship from the onset of pain in one place followed by another.

Even asymptomatic patients can have coronary disease or a silent myocardial infarction. In any admitted patient with multiple background risk factors for atherosclerosis, it is worth doing simple tests such as an electrocardiogram (ECG).

1.3 Dyspnoea

Dyspnoea or shortness of breath is another common cardiac symptom. It can be a symptom of heart failure, myocardial infarction or valvular disease. Symptoms to illicit with patients who present with dyspnoea include:

1. **Orthopnoea** (difficulty in breathing when lying flat) —

    a) 'Do you need to sleep propped up to avoid breathlessness?' Sleeping on more than two pillows may be significant. **Beware** though that orthopnoea can also occur in obese persons and people suffering from lung disorders, and that patients with back pain may also choose to sleep on several pillows.
    b) 'What happens to your breathing if you lie flat?'

2. **Paroxysmal nocturnal dyspnoea (PND)** —

    - 'Do you wake up in the night, gasping for breath, which can be relieved by sitting up or getting out of bed?'

Orthopnoea and PND are two key symptoms of heart failure. Difficulty in breathing is often worse when patients are lying flat because fluid otherwise pooled in the lower limbs returns to the heart, which backs up into the lungs.

The **onset** of dyspnoea often gives a clue as to whether the cause is cardiac or non-cardiac in origin:

- Did it come on suddenly? (Consider pulmonary embolism/ myocardial infarction.) Or did it come on gradually? (As in angina, heart failure, chronic obstructive pulmonary disease [COPD], pneumonia, or asthma.)
- Has it been getting worse?

It is important to ascertain the **severity** of dyspnoea which gives you a clinical indication of the severity of the disease. Although it is traditional to ask patients how far they can walk before they become short of breath, when this has been studied formally, it has been found to be unrelated to patients' true exercise capacity, even after correcting for their perception of distance.

To quantify the severity of dyspnoea, the **New York Heart Association (NYHA)** classification can be used:

Class 1: able to perform ordinary activities
Class 2: dyspnoea on ordinary activity, but not at rest
Class 3: dyspnoea on minimal exertion
Class 4: dyspnoea at rest

- How many flights of stairs can you climb before becoming breathless?
- Do you get short of breath at rest?

To Impress!

Save time by asking key questions:
To distinguish between a patient in Class 1 and 2:

- If you were walking along with other people of the same age and sex, do they generally have to slow down for you? Or do you keep up with them? If they keep up, they are in **Class 1**.

To distinguish between Class 2 and 3:

- When you move around from room to room at home on the same level, do you get breathless or fatigued? If yes, they are in **Class 3**. If not, they are in **Class 2**.

Class 4 should be easy to identify!

Beware: Some patients may have limited exercise tolerance due to arthritis or other conditions. See if they can tell you what symptom is actually limiting them.

1.4 Palpitations

Palpitations can be a very difficult symptom to investigate. The word 'palpitation' means the *abnormal* awareness of the hear beating in the chest, and again may mean different things to different people. Some patients feel that their heart is beating abnormally fast or slow. Other patients are aware that their heart is beating irregularly. A third group feel the heart is beating at a normal rate and regularly, but simply more intensely without good reason. It is important to identify what the patient means by palpitations. It can be helpful to ask the patient to tap out the rate and rhythm on the table. Patients with genuine significant arrhythmias are keen to do so. Patients with very brief and non-specific palpitations often decline to even try.

Some of the key questions that will help you differentiate the cause of the palpitation include:

- Is it brought on by worry?
- Does it occur on exercise or when you're excited?
- Do you notice it mainly when you're lying down? These features suggest a benign cause.
- Does it feel as though your heart drops or misses a beat? This suggests atrial or ventricular ectopics.
- Do the palpitations have an abrupt start or end? Many minutes to hours of palpitations with an abrupt start or end suggests significant pathology.

The ectopic beat is early, and followed by a compensatory pause, leading to an increase in diastolic filling time, and thus the subsequent normal beat is more forceful.

Has the patient had a 24-hour monitor/ECG? Don't forget the non-cardiac causes which are important to exclude in your history. These include:

- Drugs — that is, caffeine, nicotine, cocaine and any sympathomimetic, although remember they can both trigger pathological arrhythmias and cause simple sinus tachycardia.
- Metabolic disorders — anaemia, hyperthyroidism, and phaeochromocytoma (rare).

1.5 Syncope

Syncope can be defined as the temporary impairment of consciousness due to cerebral ischaemia. Taking an account of the attack can be divided into **three** key parts:

1) What happened *before* the faint?

   - Did you have any warning before the faint?
   - Were there any specific triggers? For example, standing up? Passing urine? Cold? The presence of a precipitant suggests a non-cardiac cause.

2) What happened *during* the faint?

   - Discover whether there were any eye witnesses. If so, obtain an eye witness account.
   - Was there any jerking, tongue biting, or incontinence? These are features of epilepsy but can occur with prolonged cardiac syncope.
   - How long did it last?

3) What happened *after* the faint?
   In general, cardiac causes of syncope involve a loss of consciousness for 1–2 minutes with complete recovery in seconds to minutes with no subsequent confusion.

   The common causes of cardiac syncope are:

   - structural heart disease leading to obstruction to outflow, i.e. seen in any of the valvular stenoses, for example, aortic stenosis and hypertrophic obstructive cardiomyopathy
   - arrhythmias such as atrial fibrillation, supraventricular tachycardias or ventricular tachycardia/fibrillation
   - pulmonary artery hypertension (rare).

Stokes Adams attack describes a transient bradycardia, a decrease in cardiac output and loss of consciousness in which there is no warning.

The patient becomes pale and drops to the floor. This can occur in any position and was originally used to describe the consequences of intermittent heart block.

Other commonly described syncopal events include vasovagal attacks, situational and postural hypotension. Vasovagal attacks are provoked by pain, fear, emotion, prolonged standing and warm environments. The response is due to **vasodilatation** and/or **bradycardia**. It doesn't occur lying down. The patient may experience preceding nausea; sweatiness and dizziness then fall to the floor and lose consciousness for 1–2 minutes.

Situational syncope is associated with specific triggers such as coughing and micturition. Postural hypotension is common in the elderly and causes dizziness or collapse on standing from lying or sitting position. This is due to inadequate reflex vasoconstriction. This response can be exacerbated if the patient is on anti-hypertensives or anti-anginals.

Don't forget to consider neurological causes such as epilepsy — that is why an eye-witness account is important (to report tongue biting, urinary incontinence, confusion, and so on). Lastly, don't forget metabolic causes such as hypoglycaemia, and drug-induced syncope (for example, blood pressure medications!).

1.6 Oedema

Peripheral oedema is the accumulation of fluid in the body's tissues. It can be divided into two types: non-pitting and pitting oedema. In non-pitting oedema the skin cannot be indented by external pressure and is due to reduced lymphatic drainage or thyroid disease. Heart failure causes pitting oedema, which is due to an increase in venous pressure secondary to ineffective pumping of the right side of the heart, together with salt and water retention. It characteristically affects both legs, often worsens as the day progresses, and is more severe the higher up the body it is located. The table below summarises a simple way to remember the causes of peripheral oedema:

Table 1.1 Causes of non-pitting and pitting oedema

Non-pitting oedema	Pitting oedema
Hypothyroidism (mucopolysaccharide deposition) Impaired lymph drainage • surgical, radiation, malignant infiltration, infectious (filariasis), congenital (Milroy's disease) Increased capillary permeability • angio-oedema	*Usually bilateral* High venous pressures • heart failure, renal failure, excessive IV fluids, steroids Low albumin states • liver failure, nephrotic syndrome, protein losing enteropathy Vasodilatation • drugs: dihydropyridines (amlodipine) and alpha-blockers (doxazosin) *Unilateral* Deep vein thrombosis Local infection, including burns

1.7 Assessment of Cardiac Risk Factors

Once you have obtained a thorough history of each of the symptoms above, a thorough assessment of the patient's cardiac risk factors can help to support or counter your diagnosis. You will be expected to be able to rattle off the list of risk factors without hesitation and to have asked the patient about each one. The greater the number of cardiac risk factors present, the greater their risk of a cardiac event.

> Remember to avoid using jargon and stick to simple terminology the patient will understand.

1.7.1 *Previous cardiac history*

Start with asking about any previous cardiac history.

- Have you had any cardiac events before?
- If so, were the symptoms similar to the current ones? What happened on that occasion, that is, what tests were performed and what were the results?
- Have you had any previous interventional procedures such as a balloon angioplasty, stent insertion or coronary artery bypass surgery (CABG)? When did you have these procedures (dates)?

1.7.2 *Hypertension*

In patients with high blood pressure, ask about duration as an indication of severity. The longer the history of hypertension, the greater the likelihood of cardiovascular disease. (See the *Hypertension* section in Chapter 4 *Commonly Encountered Patients* for more information.)

- How long have you had high blood pressure for?
- What blood pressure medications have been tried before? (Why were they stopped?)
- What blood pressure medications are you currently taking?
- Do you measure your blood pressure at home?
- What are your recent blood pressure readings?

1.7.3 *Diabetes*

Don't just say ask if they have diabetes, find out roughly what age they were diagnosed, whether they went straight to insulin therapy, the duration of their disease and severity. There are two types of diabetes. Type 1 typically presents in childhood/youth and is treated immediately with insulin. Type 2 typically is of adult onset, commonly associated with obesity and often treated with diet and

HbA1c is a molecule formed when glucose is attached to haemoglobin in the blood. As haemoglobin circulates in the blood for 8–12 weeks, measurement of HbA1c gives an indication of the average blood glucose in a patient over the last 8–12 weeks.

tablets first. Look for the presence of end organ damage to eyes, nerves and kidneys.

- Have you got any problems with your eyes or kidneys?
- Do you get pins and needles in your hands or feet?

Finding out whether or not the patient is insulin dependent can give you an idea as to the stage. Patients with diabetes have a two to four-fold increase in relative risk of developing coronary heart disease. Aim to keep the blood glucose values between 4 and 6 mmol/l and HbA1c < 6%.

- Do you measure your blood sugar at home?
- If so, what is your usual range?

1.7.4 *Hypercholesterolaemia*

Often patients won't know if they have high cholesterol, therefore it is quite useful to ask if the patient is on any cholesterol-lowering medication instead. Occasionally, there may be evidence of familial hypercholesterolaemia (a fairly rare group of severe genetic disease).

Familial hypercholesterolaemia is defined by two criteria in the patient — NOT the family!

1) Total cholesterol concentration >7.5 mmol/l, or Low Density Lipoprotein (LDL) cholesterol >4.9 mmol/l.
2) Presence of tendon xanthoma or genetic mutation of **LDL receptor/apoB-100** in 1st/2nd degree relative.

1.7.5 *Smoking*

- Do you smoke? If so, how many cigarettes do you smoke a day?
- Have you tried to stop smoking? Have you sought any specialist advice on how to stop smoking?
- If you are an ex-smoker, how long ago did you give up?

Pack years

Textbooks and tutorials often teach you to calculate the number of pack years that a patient has smoked. You will notice experienced consultants rarely actually elicit this data in practice and certainly never present it. There are two reasons for this. Firstly, the critical distinction to make is the division of patients into three groups — never smoked, ex-smoker and current smoker. This is because the ex-smokers and current smokers have a substantially elevated cardiovascular risk compared to the non-smokers. The extent of this elevation is relatively easy to judge from the age of the patient if you assume most patients start smoking in their teens. It saves time, when time is limited, not to get into the ups and downs of the patient's cigarette consumption over the years.

> The *pack year* assumes a standard pack of cigarettes has 20 cigarettes, therefore 1 pack year is equal to a patient smoking 20 cigarettes a day for a year. You can easily calculate this by this formula:
>
> $$\text{Pack years} = \frac{\text{number of cigarettes per day} \times \text{no. of years}}{20}$$

Secondly, the 'current smoker' group is vital to identify because these patients are targets for aggressive intervention. There is good evidence to show that patients who are offered advice and counselling on smoking cessation have higher odds of quitting than those without any help.

1.7.6 *Alcohol*

Small amounts of alcohol, around 1 unit per day, are consistently associated with reduced cardiac event rates for reasons that are less clear. Higher amounts of alcohol, however, can cause hypertension,

> **One unit of alcohol *equals***
> - Small glass of wine
> - Half a pint of normal strength beer
> - Single 25 mls shot of spirit

cardiomyopathy and atrial fibrillation. Ask about weekly alcohol consumption:

- How much alcohol do you drink a week? In units?
- Is this in the form of beer? Spirits? Wine? Other?

Try to quantify consumption as much as possible (see above). Keeping their alcohol consumption below the recommended limits, of up to 21 units per day for men and up to 14 units per day for women, is advisable.

1.7.7 *Family history*

Family history of cardiovascular disease (CVD) and or stroke, especially present in first degree relatives under the age of 65 in males and 55 in females, increases a patient's risk of heart disease by 1.5.

In addition to the five major risk factors discussed, physical inactivity, obesity and a high fat and high salt diet are also risk factors, although less easily quantifiable. The drug history may also highlight any medical problems the patient may have forgotten to tell you

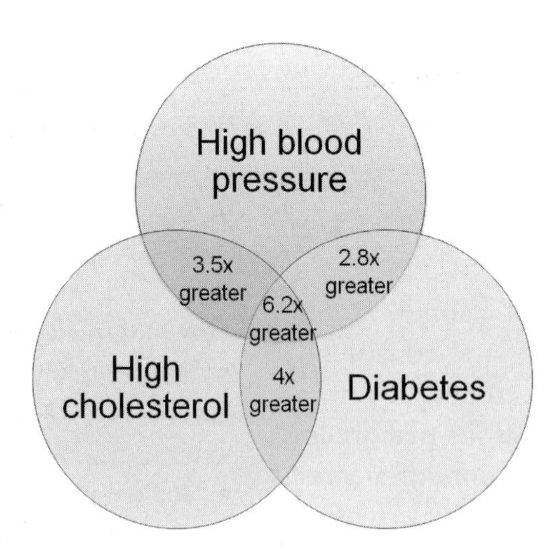

Figure 1.1 Combinational effect of each additional risk factor on cardiovascular risk

about, for example, the patient may have neglected to tell you about their hypothyroidism as they have become so accustomed to it but this can be easily picked up when the patient tells you that they take thyroxine regularly.

1.8 Social Circumstances

Don't forget the implications of the symptoms and the disease to the patients.

- What physical activity do you need to do for your work?

A myocardial infarction may cost a construction worker his job but not an office worker. What family support or responsibility does the patient have? What physical activity could the patient manage at home prior to the disease? This will help work out a realistic goal for post-discharge rehabilitation.

1.9 Implications in Primary Care

Primary prevention of cardiovascular disease in the community, even in apparently healthy individuals, is increasingly practiced. In the UK, all adults over the age of 40 undergo a comprehensive cardiovascular risk assessment in primary care once every five years. Many risk assessment models exist including the Framingham equation, Sheffield risk tables, the European coronary risk chart and the New Zealand risk assessment tool. The coronary risk prediction chart is the one recommended by the joint British societies and is based on assessment of all the risk factors including ethnicity, smoking, family history, weight, blood pressure and lipid levels. It stratifies patients according to their percentage risk over a ten-year period. These charts are useful in deciding the degree of intervention necessary, that is, simple lifestyle measures or initiating drug therapy with aspirin, anti-hypertensives and lipid lowering medications. However, the disadvantages of these charts are that they underestimate the risk in some ethnic groups and also in diabetics, patients with renal failure and inherited dyslipidaemias.

(See the joint British societies' risk prediction chart: http://www.bhsoc.org/Cardiovascular_Risk_Prediction_Chart.stm.)

- Low risk patients (green area) = calculated cardiovascular risk <10% over the next ten years.
- Intermediate risk patients (orange area) = cardiovascular risk between 10–20% in the next ten years.
- High risk patients (red area) = cardiovascular risk over 20% in the next ten years. These patients should be targeted and treated to prevent disease progression.

1.10 Examination of a Patient

Introduce yourself to the patient, explain what you would like to do and gain their permission. By shaking the patient's hand, you are not only being friendly, but also have the opportunity to assess his/her peripheral circulation.

Remember to be systematic in your approach to the patient:

general → hands → BP → neck → face → chest → oedema → finish

Adequately expose the patient's chest and position the patient at 45 degrees.

1.10.1 *General examination*

Stand at the end of the bed and briefly observe the patient's general condition. Does the patient look well or do they look unwell? Are there any devices by the bedside that would give you clues such as inhalers, cardiac monitor, external pacing, or walking aids? Does the patient look in pain or in respiratory distress? Does the patient have any dysmorphic features that may allude to an underlying congenital heart disease, for example:

- **Down's syndrome** — look for upslanting palpebral fissures, bilateral epicanthal folds (almond shaped eyes), protruding tongue and low set ears.

- **Marfan's syndrome** — tall stature, abnormally long and slender limbs (arachnodactyly).
- **Turner's syndrome** — short stature, webbing of the neck, low set ears.

Mechanical prosthetic valves can sometimes be heard from the end of the bed!

As part of your general examination, 'without touching the patient, examine the chest in a swift and focused manner for:

- Scars and external devices
  - A midline sternotomy scar could indicate a previous coronary artery bypass graft (CABG) or valve replacement.
  - A lateral thoracotomy scar could indicate mitral valve surgery.
  - A subclavicular scar and bump under the skin could indicate pacemaker/automated implantable cardiac defibrillator (AICD).
  - Vein harvesting scars on legs and radial artery harvesting scars could be a sign of bypass surgery.

With the introduction of minimally invasive interventional techniques, patients who have had angiography or other interventions may only have a small scar in the groin crease (usually the right) which you are unlikely to see. Antecubital fossa brachial artery scars are more likely to be observed.

1.10.2 *Hands*

Take your patient's hands. Warm hands suggest adequate perfusion (unless the patient is pyrexial). Start by looking at the fingertips.

Look for *clubbing* which can be described in four stages:

1. Increased fluctuancy of nail bed
2. Loss of nail bed angle
3. Increased longitudinal curvature of nail
4. Drum stick appearance of the nail caused by expansion of the terminal phalanx.

To detect clubbing, ask the patient to hold the nails of both index fingers, facing each other. In the absence of clubbing, a diamond-shaped space can be seen, caused by the angulation of both nail beds. In patients with clubbing, the diamond shape is obliterated.

The cardiac causes of clubbing can be remembered by **ABC**:

- **A**trial myxoma (rare)
- **B**acterial endocarditis (subacute)
- **C**yanotic congenital heart disease.

However, you would be expected to know a few non-cardiac causes of clubbing. Use the following mnemonic to help you remember both cardiac and non-cardiac causes:

- congenital *Cyanotic* heart disease
- **L**ung abscess, fibrosis
- **U**lcerative colitis/Crohn's disease
- **B**iliary cirrhosis
- **B**ronchiectasis
- **I**nfective endocarditis
- **N**eoplastic disease, for example, lung cancer and Hodgkin's disease
- **G**astrointestinal malabsorption.

Look closely at the nails also for signs of bacterial endocarditis characterised by splinter haemorrhages (which can also occur due to trauma, for example, in manual labourers), Janeway lesions and Osler nodes (see section on *Endocarditis in Chapter 2: Bedside teaching*). A simple thing to comment on (which shows you are observant) is tar staining on the fingers, as smoking is a risk factor for cardiovascular disease.

Look for hypercholesterolaemic deposits in the skin as yellow nodules known as tendon and palmar xanthomas.

1.10.3 *Radial pulse*

Feel for the pulse for at least 15 seconds and comment on the rate and rhythm. Is it slow (bradycardic) or fast (tachycardic), regular or irregular? A congenital condition known as coarctation of the aorta is where there is a narrowing somewhere along the descending aorta. This manifests as radial-radial delay or radial-femoral delay which can be detected by feeling pulses in two places simultaneously. Most aortic coarctations are distal to both subclavian arteries so only the radio-femoral delay is abnormal.

1.10.4 *Blood pressure*

Moving up the arm in your examination ensures you don't miss the blood pressure. Comment on it, if it's available, otherwise say you would like to measure it. (See the *Appendix* on how to measure blood pressure for tips.) The pulse pressure is the difference between the systolic and diastolic pressures. The pulse pressure is typically wide in aortic regurgitation and although many textbooks say it is narrow in aortic stenosis, this is simply not the case and patients with aortic stenosis often have normal pulse pressures. There is also a phenomenon known as **pulsus paradoxus** where there is a drop in systolic blood pressure during inspiration of 10 mmHg. It is something you might get asked about on ward rounds as it is associated with pericardial constriction, tamponade and severe asthma. Look also for **pulsus alternans**, the alternating of strong and weak beats sometimes seen in severe left ventricular systolic impairment. Comment on any postural blood pressure changes. A postural drop in blood pressure is defined as a drop in systolic BP of >15 mmHg or a diastolic drop of >10 mmHg after a patient stands from lying down.

1.10.5 *Neck*

There are two important structures in the neck in the cardiovascular examination, the jugular venous pulse (JVP) and the carotid pulse. The internal jugular vein (IJV) gives an indirect measure of the pressure in the right atrium (RA) and provides some information about cardiac function — this is because there are no valves between the RA and IJV. The IJV enters the neck just behind the mastoid process, passes deep to the sternocleidomastoid muscle (SCM) and then runs

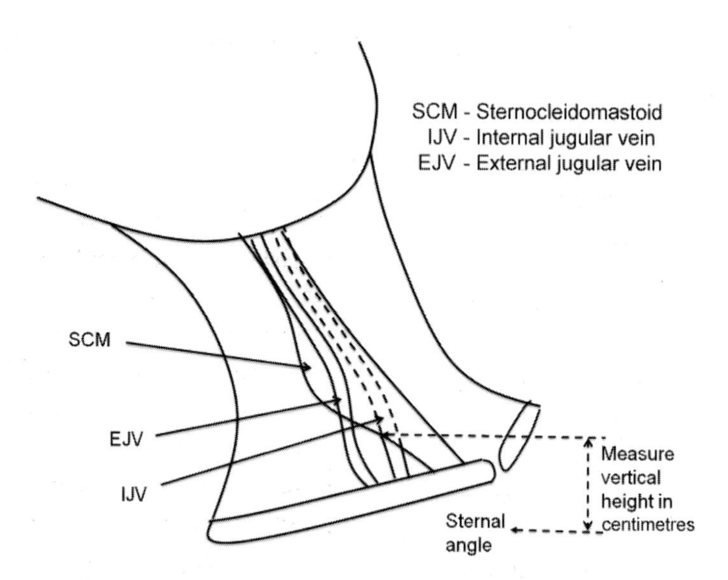

Figure 1.2 Measuring the JVP

between the sternal and clavicular heads of the SCM before entering the thorax. The IJV itself is not visible.

To measure the JVP, sit the patient at a 45 degree angle, with the neck muscles relaxed and head turned slightly to the left. Look for diffuse pulsations. The JVP is the vertical height of the pulse in the IJV above the sternal angle. The normal JVP is <4 cm.

A common question you are likely to encounter is how you would differentiate between the JVP and the carotid pulse.

The six key features to distinguish JVP from carotid artery:

The JVP:

1) pulsation is easily obliterated by finger pressure
2) has two pulsations for each single arterial pulse
3) is much weaker in force (impalpable)
4) varies with respiration
5) varies with position
6) rises transiently with pressure on the liver (hepatojugular reflux) or on the abdomen (abdominojugular reflux).

Two important things to note about the JVP are the **height** and **waveform**.

A *raised JVP* can be a sign of:

- fluid overload
- right-sided heart failure
- SVC obstruction
- constrictive pericarditis.

> **To Impress!**
> **Positive hepatojugular reflux** sign is not simply the elevation of the JVP on hepatic compression as this occurs in everyone but rather that the JVP **remains** elevated for a 15 second compression. This is because the RV is unable to pump out the increased venous return — a sign of RV heart failure.

In constrictive pericarditis, an elevated JVP is characteristically associated with a paradoxical rise in inspiration — known as **Kussmaul's sign**.

To understand waveform abnormalities, it is important to understand the actual waveform. The waveform corresponds to the changes in right atrial pressure. There are two peaks and two descents.

The normal JVP goes down in systole (x descent). Systole starts with the brief c wave and then proceeds with the x descent as the right atrial floor moves down as a result of right ventricular contraction. Late in systole, the veins start to fill the atrium faster than its capacity is being increased by ventricular contraction and so there is a passive accommodation of blood and therefore increase in pressure which corresponds to the v wave.

The abnormalities can be divided broadly into a wave and v wave abnormalities.

'A wave' abnormalities

An *absent a wave* (and so the JVP rate is similar to the pulse rate) indicates no atrial contraction and occurs in atrial fibrillation. A *large a wave* is hard to diagnose clinically but in an exam you need to understand

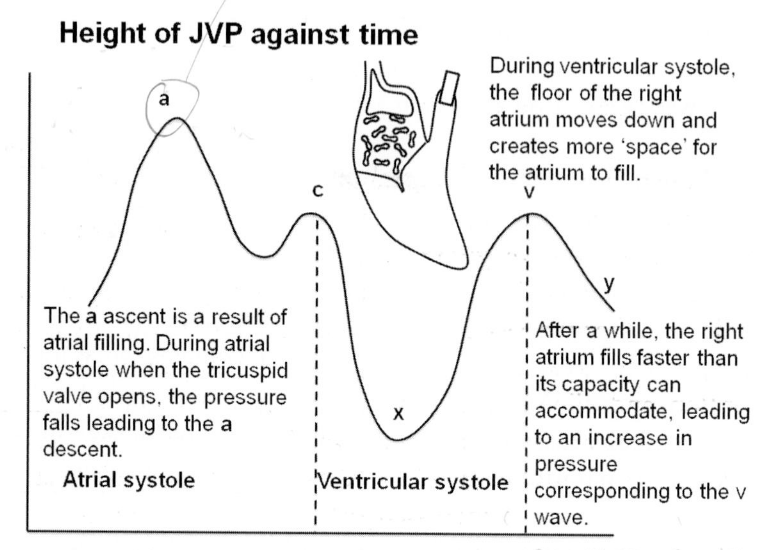

a wave: **a**trial systole
c wave: **c**losure of tricuspid valve
x descent: drop in atrial pressure during ventricular systole
v wave: passive **v**enous filling of atria with closed tricuspid valve
y descent: tricuspid valve opening

Figure 1.3 Height of JVP against time

that this occurs when the right atrium is contracting against resistance, that is, in pulmonary hypertension and pulmonary stenosis. *Cannon 'a' waves* are caused by a right atrium contracting intermittently against a closed tricuspid valve, which occurs in complete heart block.

V wave abnormalities

In tricuspid regurgitation, right ventricular contraction does not only pull down the floor of the right atrium, but also ejects a lot of blood into the right atrium, hence the JVP goes up. This is **not** passive venous filling, so it is not a large v wave. In fact, it starts at the c wave and continues to the end of the v wave. Its proper name is a giant *CV* wave, and can be thought of as an upside down x descent. The JVP may be so high in the neck that it can only be seen by looking behind the ear — a large v wave can cause the ears to waggle!

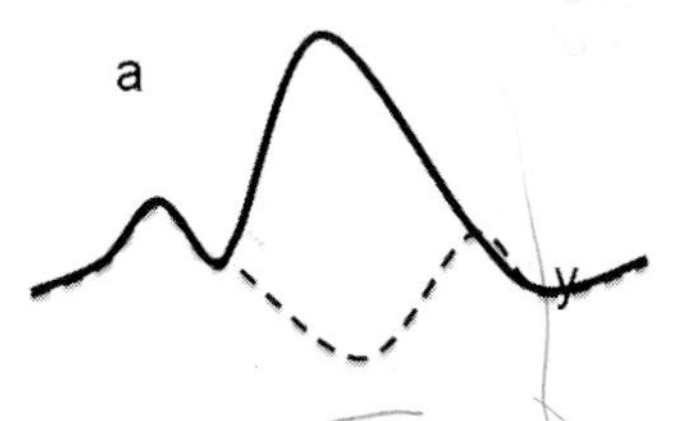

Figure 1.4 Giant CV wave

In practice, it is difficult to pick up a JVP *waveform* abnormality, and valvular heart disease is rarely diagnosed on the basis of an abnormal JVP waveform. However, it is important to recognise whether the JVP is raised or not, and to know what conditions are associated with the different waveform abnormalities both for written and clinical examinations. Tricuspid regurgitation and atrial fibrillation are two common examination cases. In addition, there is some evidence that an elevated JVP in patients with heart failure is associated with an increased risk of hospital admission, death and subsequent hospitalisation for heart failure.

The carotid pulse

The carotid artery can be found by placing the thumb gently on the trachea and sliding the thumb laterally until it hits the sternocleidomastoid where the carotid pulse should be palpable. Four things should be noted about the pulse — the *rate*, *rhythm*, *volume* and *character*. The rate and rhythm should already have been assessed when examining the radial pulse. The volume and character should be assessed at the carotid rather than the radial as it is closer to the heart.

The volume may be:

- **low** — in shock and heart failure, or
- **large** — in aortic regurgitation, vasodilatation (exercise, fever).

There are several distinct character pulses:

- **slow rising** occurs in aortic stenosis
- **collapsing pulse** occurs in regurgitation
- **bisferens pulse**, where two distinct systolic peaks are present, characteristic of aortic regurgitation and stenosis.

Don't forget to listen for carotid bruits — ask patients to hold their breath whilst simultaneously listening with the bell of the stethoscope (it's a good idea to hold your breath with the patient as it reminds you how long you're asking them to do this). The presence of carotid bruits can suggest local disease or radiation from elsewhere, that is, in aortic stenosis. Ask yourself whether the patient has any other clinical features of peripheral arterial disease and remember in an exam situation to at least offer to palpate peripheral pulses at the end of the examination.

1.10.6 *Face*

Start from top down — look at the eyes for evidence of cataracts, which can be a result of diabetes or hypertensive retinopathy. A pale conjunctiva is indicative of anaemia. Pallor with jaundice suggests haemolytic anaemia. Lid lag and exophthalmos indicates thyroid disease. Look for the presence of corneal arcus, a grey opaque line surrounding the cornea and xanthelasmata which are yellow fatty deposits commonly found around the eyes. Both of these signs are associated with raised cholesterol levels.

Jaundice can signify haemolysis which can result as a complication of prosthetic valves. Central cyanosis on the tongue can indicate congenital heart disease.

1.10.7 *Praecordium*

Examine for scars particularly at the apex where they can be easily missed. Feel the position of the apex by placing the palm of your right hand over the left chest wall: is it displaced? If so, where — for example, laterally? Downwards? Be specific. The normal position of the apex is in the fifth intercostals space, mid-clavicular line. Abnormal characteristics of the apex beat can be described as 1) heaving, which occurs in volume

> **Top tip:** When you know the apex beat is abnormal but do not know if it is heaving or thrusting say *'forceful'*.

overloaded conditions like mitral and aortic regurgitation; 2) thrusting, which occurs in pressure overloaded conditions like aortic stenosis.

Volume overload — conditions: mitral or aortic regurgitation
— leads to dilatation of the LV → displacement of the apex
— detectable on Chest X-ray (CXR) if severe

Pressure overload — conditions: aortic stenosis, hypertension
— leads to concentric hypertrophy of the LV → thicker LV wall (hypertrophy)
— detectable on ECG (sometimes).

Only echocardiography is truly reliable for detecting these.

If the apex is displaced, this is due to either mediastinal shift or dilatation of the heart:

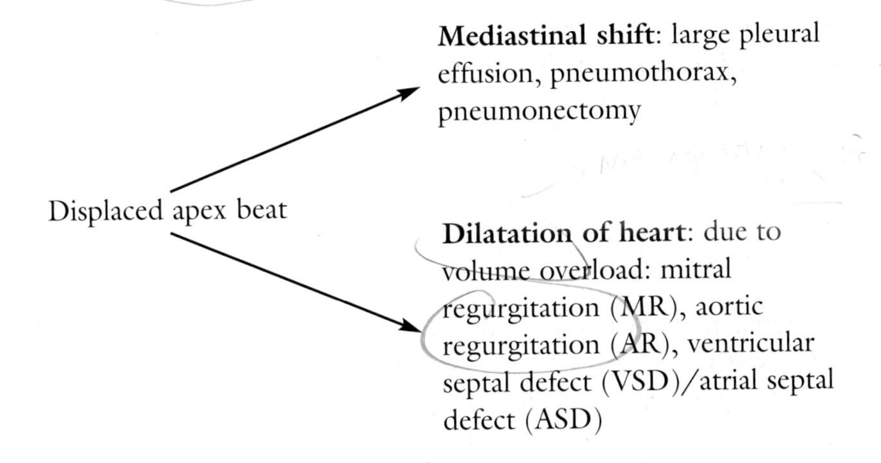

To feel for thrills, keep your hand over the apex and then palpate over both sides of the sternum. *A thrill is a palpable murmur — it feels like a purring cat.* Now feel for a right ventricular (RV) heave by placing your hand in the left parasternal position. A RV heave is a palpable beat and suggests RV enlargement, which can occur in cor pulmonale or pulmonary stenosis.

Cor pulmonale is right ventricular failure secondary to chronic pulmonary hypertension which can be a result of lung disease, pulmonary vascular disorders, neuromuscular and skeletal diseases.

Stenosis of the **pulmonary artery** causes increased pressure in the right ventricle and leads to hypertrophy.

1.10.8 *Auscultation of the heart*

Most stethoscopes have a bell and diaphragm. When auscultating, you are listening for:

- normal heart sounds
- added heart sounds, that is, murmurs (due to turbulent blood flow) or a third or fourth heart sound.

The **bell** is best used for low pitched sounds:

- diastolic murmurs, for example, mitral stenosis
- third and fourth heart sounds.

The **diaphragm** is better for detecting higher pitched sounds:

- normal heart sounds
- systolic murmurs
- aortic regurgitation.

With the patient sitting at 45 degrees first listen at the apex, tricuspid, pulmonary and aortic areas with the bell and then again with the diaphragm. Place your thumb on the patient's carotid pulse whilst auscultating the heart sounds — this helps to differentiate the first (S1) and second (S2) heart sounds and any murmurs.

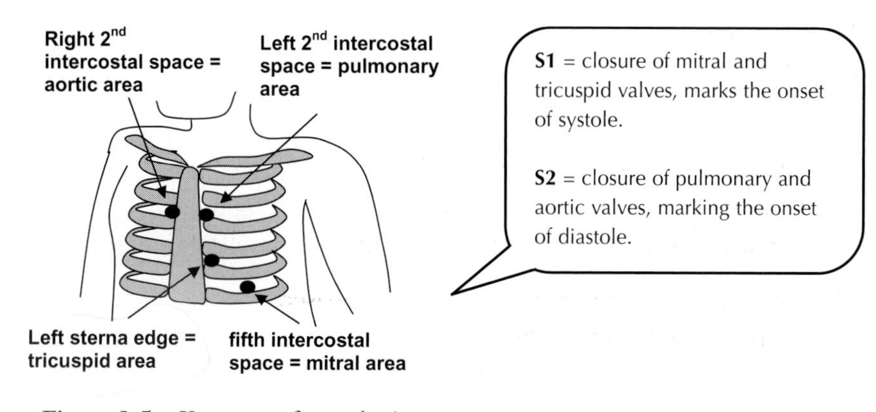

Figure 1.5 Key areas of auscultation

Splitting of the second heart sound:

S2 has two components: A2 (closure of aortic valve) and P2 (closure of pulmonary valve). In most people S2 is heard as one sound. However, it is normal to hear a split S2 on inspiration in the young.

Why is this? — On inspiration, intrathoracic pressures drop which leads to an increase in venous return to the right heart. This in turn leads to a delay in right heart emptying and so the pulmonary valve remains open for longer, closing later (after the aortic valve).

Abnormal splitting:

Wide 'fixed' splitting in atrial septal defect (ASD): S2 remains split in inspiration and expiration.

Wide 'physiological' splitting in right bundle branch block (RBBB): S2 is split in expiration, but more so in inspiration.

Reverse splitting in left bundle branch block (LBBB): S2 is split in expiration and not inspiration.

Roll the patient onto the left side and listen at the apex for mitral murmurs and then in the axilla for any radiation of the murmur. Sit the patient up and leaning forwards. This time listen in the aortic and tricuspid areas with the diaphragm. If a murmur is heard, determine the timing (that is, systolic or diastolic). Ask the patient to take a deep breath in and hold their breath. Then get the patient to take a deep breath in, out and hold their breath at the end of the expiration. **R**ight-sided murmurs are louder on **i**nspiration and **l**eft-sided murmurs louder on **e**xpiration — **RILE**. For a more detailed description on murmurs see Chapter 2 *Bedside Teaching*. Listen to the bases of the lungs for bilateral crepitations (as in pulmonary oedema) or reduced air entry and dullness (pleural effusions). Feel for sacral oedema.

To complete examination:

- **Check the abdomen for**: an enlarged liver (right-heart failure), a pulsatile liver edge occurs in tricuspid regurgitation or midline pulsatile mass (aortic aneurysm).
- **Check the legs and sacrum** for pitting oedema: use a finger to gently but firmly push against a bony surface and look to see if the indentation remains.
- **Dip the urine for haematuria** (in infective endocarditis), glucose (diabetes — a risk factor for cardiovascular disease).

1.11 Worked Example

Below is a worked example to highlight the key points in clerking and presenting a patient complaining of chest pain:

Student: Good morning. Can I check that I have come to the right person? What is your name?

Patient: My name is Mr. R.

Student: My name is X. I'm one of the student doctors and I would like to ask you some questions. Is that alright?

> Greet the patient, introduce yourself and explain what you intend to do.

Patient: Yes, that's fine.

Student: How old are you?

Patient: 72.

Student: Are you retired now?

Patient: Yes. Six years now. I used to be an electrician.

Step 1 Presenting Complaint

Student: What brought you into hospital?

Patient: Well, I just wasn't feeling right yesterday.

Student: In what way?

Patient: I had this discomfort across my chest.

> Use open-ended questions and avoid too many leading questions.

Student: Where was this discomfort on your chest?

Patient: Here on the left side.

Student: Did it spread anywhere else?

Patient: Not really, but I did start to get a heaviness in my left hand.

Student: Can you describe the chest discomfort?

Patient: It was like a pressure — like someone sitting on my chest.

> Use of **SOCRATES** questions.

Student: When did it start?

Patient: Probably about 1pm. I was walking the dog and had just reached the hill.

Student: What did you do then?

Patient: I carried on walking for a few minutes but the pain became unbearable, so I stopped and sat on one of the park benches.

Student: Did this help?

Patient: A little. It definitely helped me get my breath back.

Student: Were you feeling short of breath at the time?

Patient: Yes. That's strange for me — I never get short of breath when I'm walking the dog.

Student: Going back to the chest discomfort, at its worst, how severe was the pain on a scale of one to ten, where ten is the worst discomfort that you've ever felt?

Patient: I'd say about nine.

Student: What did you do after sitting on the bench?

Patient: Well after ten minutes, the pain was still there so I got up and went back home. My wife said I looked really pale and called the ambulance.

Student: Did you feel clammy at all?

Patient: Yes and nauseous.

> Ask about associated symptoms.

Student: Did you actually vomit?

Patient: No.

Student: Any dizziness?

Patient: No.

Student: Did you blackout at any point?

Patient: No.

Student: Did you feel your heart fluttering in your chest?

Patient: No.

Student: Do you ever get short of breath on lying flat?

Patient: No.

Student: How many pillows do you sleep with?

> If patient starts to ramble, gently guide the conversation back.

Patient: Only the one.

Student: Do you ever find that your ankles become puffy or swollen?

Patient: No, but I do often get these pains in my ankles and knees. My GP said it was probably arthritis. I hope I don't need an operation. My wife had to have her knees replaced last year.

Student: Ok, we will talk about the arthritis a bit later. Can I just clarify a few things… Going back to the chest discomfort — did anything make it better?

Patient: Not really. It only went away after I reached the hospital.

Student: Were you given anything at the hospital or by the paramedics that helped ease the pain?

Patient: Oh yes — the oxygen really helped, but I also had a tablet and a spray under my tongue.

Student: How long did you have the pain for in total?

Patient: About an hour or so.

Step 2 Cardiac Risk Factors

Student: Have you ever had this kind of discomfort before or any chest pain in the past?
Patient: No, not at all.
Student: Have you ever had a heart attack?
Patient: No, but my father has.
Student: How old was he when he had the heart attack?
Patient: He was 59 I think.
Student: Do you have **diabetes**?
Patient: No.
Student: Do you have **high blood pressure**?
Patient: Not anymore. I'm on tablets.
Student: Do you **smoke**?
Patient: No, never have done.
Student: What about your **cholesterol**?
Patient: I think my cholesterol is fine doctor.

> Risk factors for cardiovascular disease.

> Here's where you discover your patient who previously told you he didn't have high cholesterol does not have high cholesterol because he is being controlled with a statin!

Step 3 Drug History

Student: Are you on any medication?
Patient: Yes, I take a cholesterol tablet once a night and a water tablet.

Step 4 Past Medical History

Student: Have you ever been admitted to hospital before?
Patient: No, I've never been sick in my life.
Student: Have you ever had any operations?
Patient: No.
Student: Do you have any medical problems?
Patient: No.

Step 5 Social History

Student: Who do you live with?
Patient: I live with my wife.
Student: Do you live in a house? Flat?
Patient: In a house.
Student: Do you manage the stairs ok?
Patient: Yes.
Student: Do you drink any alcohol?
Patient: Yes, 2–3 pints only on Sundays.
Student: Have you ever tried recreational drugs? Such as cocaine.
Patient: Oh no, I would never touch those things.

1.12 Presenting Patients

When presenting patients, for example on a ward round, it is important to be logical and coherent. Some consultants may have specific ways in which they wish to have the information presented, but on the whole the following can be used.

1.13 Summarising Your History

In the first opening statement you should include:

- name
- age
- occupation
- sex
- *brief* presenting complaint (in patient's own words)
- any previous cardiac disease
- any cardiac risk factors.

When presenting the history, it is important to mention the relevant *positive and negative findings*. For example, in a patient in whom you suspect congestive cardiac failure you must mention whether he/she reports any orthopnoea, paroxysmal nocturnal dyspnoea (PND), or ankle swelling, and what their exercise tolerance is.

1.13.1 *An example of a presentation based on the previous history*

Student: Mr R is a 72-year old retired electrician who presented to the Emergency Department yesterday complaining of 'chest discomfort'. He has no previous history of ischaemic heart disease but his cardiac risk factors are hypertension, hypercholesterolaemia and a positive family history.

The chest pain occurred on exertion, whilst the patient was walking his dog, was not relieved by rest and lasted a total of one hour. It was located on the left of the chest and was radiating to the left arm. Associated symptoms were nausea, dyspnoea and feeling clammy. There were no palpitations, loss of consciousness or dizziness, orthopnoea or ankle swelling. With regards to cardiac risk factors he has hypertension and high cholesterol, for which he is being treated and his father suffered a myocardial infarction aged 59 years. He has not had a previous myocardial infarction, denies ischaemic heart disease and is not diabetic. He is a non-smoker, lives with his wife and is independent of his activities of daily living.

Chapter 2

Bedside Teaching

Although bedside teaching is an integral part of medical student training, it tends to be informal and haphazard, and it is sometimes difficult to gauge what information to take away in order to maximise one's experience on the wards. This section covers the common types of patients found on cardiology wards with specific hints and tips on what to look out for when examining these patients, as well as how to tackle consultant grilling in a dependable, systematic manner.

2.1 Tackling Murmurs

The patients most easily singled out for students to examine are those with murmurs as these have demonstrable signs. Everyone is quick to jump to auscultation; however, a lot of telling signs can be gained before you even place your stethoscope on the patient. Thus, always remember to start every examination the same way (refer to the section on examination of the patient in *Chapter 1 Clerking patients*). The important things to pay attention to at the end of the bed include:

- **Signs of cardiac failure**
  - Is the patient short of breath? On oxygen? Count the respiratory rate.
  - Is there any evidence of oedema?
- **Presence of chest scars**
  - A midline sternotomy scar could be due to aortic or mitral valve replacement or a coronary artery bypass graft (in which

case have a good look at the medial side of the legs and arms for vessel harvest scars).
  - Thoracotomy scars are more likely to be mitral valve scars.

- **Signs of infective endocarditis**
  - Hand signs — Osler nodes, Janeway lesions, and so on.
  - Systemic features — for example, fever.

Different trainers (and different examiners) will prefer you to do things in slightly different way. Some prefer you to present your signs as you pick them up, others prefer you to keep a mental note of the signs in your head and present at the end when you can piece all the signs together. Make sure you can do both (practice both ways). In the exam situation, *choose whichever way you prefer*. The examiner may indicate their preference, so be ready to adapt accordingly.

After inspection, start with the hands, taking a good 15 seconds' pulse and note whether the pulse is regular or irregular. Remember the character and volume of the pulse is better determined at the carotids, as the pulse at the neck lies closer to the heart. The pulse can be described as:

- **normal**
- **slow-rising** (think: aortic stenosis)
- **large volume** (think: aortic regurgitation and check for a collapsing pulse)
- textbooks also describe a double pulsation also known as a **bisferens pulse**, which is supposed to indicate mixed valvular disease. It is very unlikely that you will ever feel such a pulse, and trying to diagnose it is likely to complicate your life more than it helps.

When it comes to auscultation, it is by no means an easy feat especially when you are under pressure. Before you reach around your neck for your stethoscope, make sure to locate the apex beat by feeling the most lateral point of the thoracic wall and sweeping your fingers across the chest medially. Starting at the lateral wall ensures you do

Grades of murmurs

G1: soft murmur detectable after careful auscultation
G2: soft murmur readily evident
G3: moderate murmur
G4: loud murmur
G5: loud murmur with thrill
G6: loud murmur audible without stethoscope

not miss a displaced apex. If abnormal, identify the position, by making efforts that the examiner can see clearly, to count rib spaces, and determine the position relative to the mid-clavicular or anterior axillary lines. Textbooks describe the difference between an apex beat that is *pressure* or *volume* overloaded. *Heaving* is often used to describe the former and *thrusting* the latter. However, in the examination situation it may be less stressful not to try to distinguish these unless confident.

2.1.1 *Using the stethoscope*

S3 is due to rapid ventricular filling.

Place your stethoscope over the apex beat while feeling the carotid pulse at the same time. Listen for the heart sounds. Remember S1 corresponds to the closure of the mitral and tricuspid valves and S2 corresponds to the closure of the aortic and pulmonary valves. The first heart sound S1 should coincide with the carotid pulse. S2 follows. There may be a third heart sound — an S3 sounds like a horse's gallop or the word 'Ken-tuck-y', whereas S4 occurs just before S1 and sounds like 'Tennessee'. Listen and time any murmurs — do they occur straight after S1 or S2? Determine:

- **where** in the cycle they occur
- how **loud** the murmur is (either soft/moderate/loud, or if you prefer, a numerical grade 1–6)

It is tricky the first few times you examine a patient with a murmur but if you keep practicing, you will become familiar with the different types of murmurs.

Table 2.1 Comparing systolic and diastolic murmurs

Systolic murmur (between S1–S2) consider	**Diastolic murmur** (between S2–S1) consider
Ejection systolic murmur — aortic stenosis, atrial septal defect, hypertrophic cardiomyopathy	**Early diastolic murmur** — aortic regurgitation
Pansystolic murmur — mitral regurgitation, tricuspid regurgitation, ventral septal defect	**Mid-diastolic murmur** — mitral stenosis
Mitral regurgitation is by far the most common. Consider ventral septal defect if a young patient. Tricuspid regurgitation is usually fairly soft (because the right heart is at low pressure) and if audible is usually associated with giant systolic waves in the jugular venous pressure.	The key question to ask yourself is, 'Does the murmur start immediately at S2, or is there a gap?' Aortic regurgitation is always continuous with S2. Mitral stenosis always has a gap between S2, and the opening of the mitral valve.

2.2 Systolic Murmurs

Remember: **LEFT**-sided murmurs (that is, those concerning the aortic and mitral valve) are heard loudest when the patient is in expiration. Similarly, **RIGHT**-sided murmurs (that is, those concerning the pulmonary and tricuspid valve) are accentuated when the patient is in inspiration; **RILES** — right inspiration, left expiration.

During expiration, the whole heart, left and right, is nearer the front of the chest, which is why it is a good time to hear the soft murmurs of mitral stenosis and aortic regurgitation.

Inspiration increases the venous return to the heart and the extra blood flow across the right-sided heart valves, making the right-sided murmurs appear louder.

2.2.1 *Aortic stenosis (AS)*

This is probably one of the commonest valvular conditions you will come across on the wards and you should therefore develop a slick

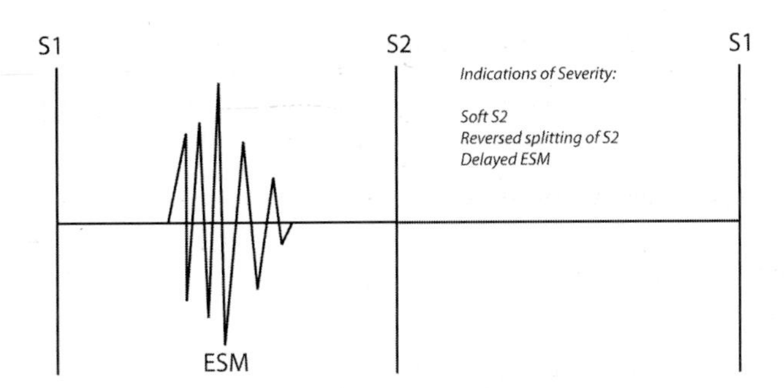

Figure 2.1 Aortic stenosis

way of examining and presenting these patients that will cover all the important points and impress your consultant. An **ejection systolic murmur (ESM)** is usually quite easy to hear. It is characterised by a crescendo-decrescendo systolic murmur that is loudest in the second intercostal space (ics) of the right sternal edge over the aortic area and is accentuated when the patient is sitting forward in *expiration*. If the ESM is louder on inspiration, it would suggest a right-sided murmur; therefore think pulmonary stenosis (much rarer than AS). Listen carefully to S2. A soft S2 signifies severe disease. Once you've established this, try to put the pieces together. Does the patient have other features consistent with AS? These include:

- slow rising regular pulse
- heaving apex beat, not displaced
- thrill in the aortic area

Check for radiation to the carotids by getting the patient to hold his/her breath while you listen with the stethoscope at the neck for a bruit. Always finish your presentation by making sure you cover the following points:

- Look for **features of infective endocarditis** and say, 'If part of the reason to examine the patient is suspicion of endocarditis, I would also:
    - dipstick the urine for protein

  - check the patient's temperature and
  - look in the eyes with a fundoscope for Roth spots (round white spots surrounded by haemorrhage).

- Look for features of **cardiac failure**.
  - Auscultate lung bases
  - Check for ankle and sacral oedema

- Look for evidence of **severity** indicated by
  - Soft S2
  - Fourth heart sound (S4)
  - Slow rising pulse
  - Delayed ejection systolic murmur-ESM (*not* the loudness)

Historically, there was a diagnosis called '**aortic sclerosis**', indicating an ESM arising from a diseased but not narrowed aortic valve. This term is now rarely used by cardiologists, who more commonly refer to the condition as a mild form of aortic stenosis.

If you are not sure whether the murmur is an ESM, it is reasonable to consider other possibilities. Other causes of a systolic murmur include:

- **Mitral regurgitation**: the distinguishing feature is a murmur of constant intensity that lasts throughout the whole of systole and can sometimes obliterate S2. Practically, it is not always that easy to distinguish and one would look for other signs to point you towards the right diagnosis, for example, a displaced thrusting apex beat, or possible atrial fibrillation (AF).
- **Ventra septal defect (VSD):** suspect particularly if your patient is young.

The commonest questions consultants will ask you with regards to a patient with AS are:

1. The symptoms a patient may present with:
   - **S**yncope
   - **A**ngina
   - **D**yspnoea

2. The commonest causes:
   - Degenerative
   - Congenital (from a biscupid valve)
   - Rheumatic

Beware as patients with Hypertrophic obstructive cardiomyopathy present with similar symptoms!

3. The investigations you would perform:
   - **Electrocardiogram (ECG)**: look for left ventricular hypertrophy
   - **Chest radiograph**: usually normal but may show evidence of cardiac failure
   - **Echocardiogram**: to calculate the valve area and velocity across the valve as an indication of severity
   - **Cardiac catheterisation** is then carried out as a prelude to surgery, to determine whether the coronary arteries need to be grafted at the same time (this turns out to be the case in about half such patients)
4. Management of such a patient:
   - **Conservative** for moderate aortic stenosis patients who are asymptomatic with regular review to detect deterioration
   - **Surgery** is recommended for patients who have a severe aortic stenosis, with peak velocity across the valve of >4 m/s, or an estimated pressure drop across the valve of >64 mm Hg, or if the patient is symptomatic. Operative mortality depends on age and frailty and is typically 2–5%

There is a low threshold for surgery in patients with AS due to the risk of syncope.

2.2.2 *Mitral regurgitation (MR)*

Another common valvular condition characterised by a **pansystolic murmur**, that is, a murmur that continues throughout the length of the systole. It is generally soft and can be accentuated with the patient

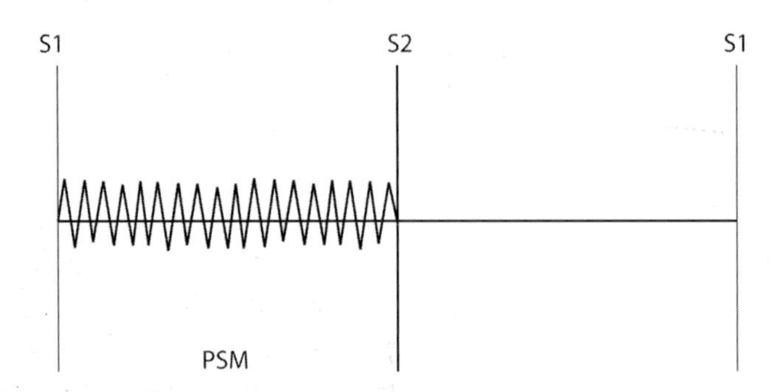

Figure 2.2 Mitral regurgitation

in the left lateral position in *expiration*. The other signs consistent with this diagnosis include:

- atrial fibrillation
- fluid overload/displaced apex beat
- thrill at apex
- **radiation to the axilla** (remember to place your stethoscope at the axilla to verify this)
- soft S1

Again as before, it is important to conclude with the following:

- look for signs of **cardiac failure**
- look for signs of **infective endocarditis**

The commonest reason to develop MR is dilation of the left ventricle, caused by heart failure of any cause.

Other than this, the main causes of MR are:

- Congenital (myxomatous or 'floppy' mitral valve)
- Acquired:
  - rheumatic
  - Marfan's syndrome, systemic lupus erythematosus
  - amyloidosis

The investigations are similar to those for AS and include:

- **ECG**: looking for p-mitrale (bifid P wave, indicates left atrial dilatation)
- **Chest radiograph**: may show cardiomegaly
- **Echocardiography**: to grade the severity of the condition and judge the impact on the left ventricle and atrium
- **Transoesophageal echocardiogram (TOE)**: to view in detail the individual cusps of the mitral valve and clearly visualise the cause, and determine whether it is a plausible case to be repaired (that is, avoiding a prosthetic valve being implanted — so no warfarin needed)
- **Catheterisation**: is often carried out in severe cases to measure pressure waveforms (and exclude coronary artery disease), and is always carried out before surgery, in case coronary artery bypass grafting is also needed.

Management can be medical or surgical. Medical therapy includes the use of diuretics and Angiotensin-Converting Enzyme (ACE) inhibitors, with warfarin added if there is atrial fibrillation. Surgery is typically valve *replacement* with a prosthesis that requires warfarin for life. Some cases of MR arising from myxomatous valves can instead be *repaired* by surgery, avoiding the need for warfarin.

2.2.3 *Tricuspid regurgitation (TR)*

Your main differential diagnosis for a **pansystolic murmur** (PSM) will be tricuspid regurgitation which is usually a result of secondary pulmonary hypertension. As this is a right-sided murmur, this PSM is heard **loudest at the tricuspid area** and is accentuated by ***inspiration***. The following features will help you to favour a diagnosis of TR over MR, although both should be in your list of differentials if you are really unsure.

- Other signs of pulmonary hypertension include loud P2 (pulmonary component of the second heart sound), right ventricular heave, a raised jugular venous pressure (JVP) with characteristic **systolic 'cv' waves**, sacral and ankle oedema (it is important to

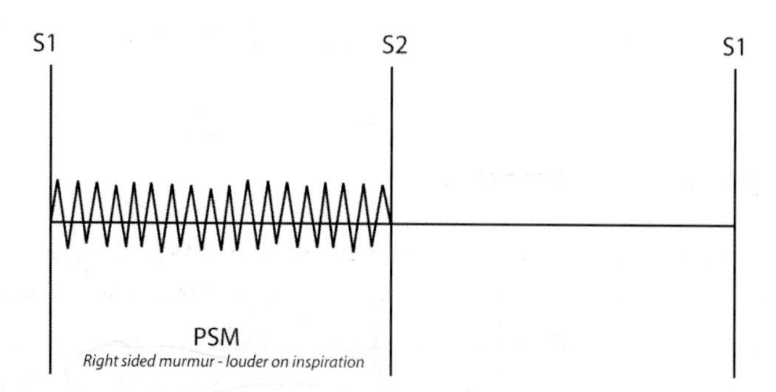

Figure 2.3 Tricuspid murmur

note that the latter three are also features of cardiac failure and fluid overload) and **pulsatile liver**

Also:

- look for signs of intravenous drug abuse
- look for signs of infective endocarditis

The causes of tricuspid regurgitation can be divided into:

- pulmonary hypertension of any cause
- left heart failure of any cause
- rarer causes including:
  - rheumatic
  - carcinoid
  - intravenous drug use

The management options are:

- medical with diuretics and ACE inhibitors
- surgical repair

2.3 Diastolic Murmurs

Diastolic murmurs are more difficult to hear as they tend to be soft. The bell of the stethoscope can be used to elicit these and should not be pressed too hard to the skin (which obliterates the bell effect).

2.3.1 *Mitral stenosis (MS)*

Observe a **malar flush** from the end of the bed. This is present in 60% of females with MS and is due to pulmonary hypertension. If you notice the patient is in atrial fibrillation (AF) when examining the pulse, keep mitral stenosis in mind and you will be sure to listen extra carefully for the soft murmur. The apex beat is said to be **tapping** in nature: this tapping is actually a very loud S1 which is palpable. On auscultation a **mid-diastolic murmur (MDM)** can be heard, loudest with the patient in the **left lateral position in expiration**. It radiates to the axilla. If sinus rhythm is noted, listen for a pre-systolic accentuation of the murmur. S1 is generally loud and there may be an **opening snap**.

Rarely, you may also hear a **Graham steel murmur** (an early diastolic murmur at the right parasternal area) which occurs due to pulmonary hypertension causing functional incompetence of the pulmonary valve.

Complete your examination by looking for evidence of

- **cardiac failure**
- **embolism**! Has the patient had a previous history of stroke?

In theory, your differential diagnosis includes an Austin Flint murmur (the appearance of a mid-diastolic murmur [MDM] in a patient with aortic regurgitation [AR], caused by the aortic

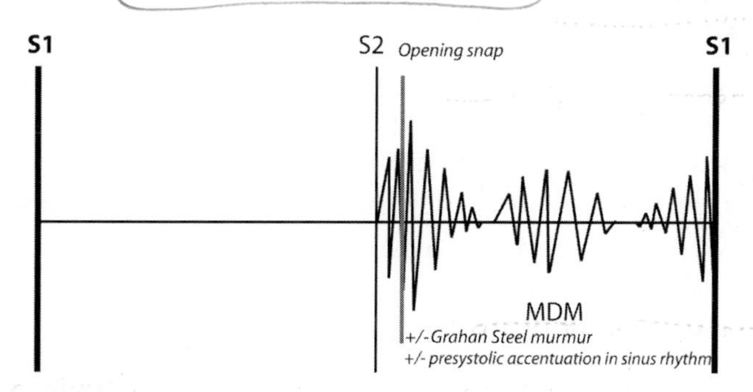

Figure 2.4 Mitral stenosis

regurgitation flow running down the anterior surface of a normal mitral valve and creating reverberations in the mitral inflow) and left atrial myxoma.

The cause of MS is usually **rheumatic**.

The investigations are familiar to you by now and include:

- **ECG**
- **chest radiograph**: looking for an enlarged left atrium
- **echocardiography**
- **+/– catheterisation**

Management:

- **Medical**: diuretics; if there is atrial fibrillation: warfarin (and digoxin)
- **Surgical**:
  - valvuloplasty
  - valvulotomy or valve replacement

valvuloplasty = percutaneous repair

valvulotomy = direct cutting of the valve

2.3.2 *Aortic regurgitation (AR)*

This is another fluid overloaded condition and usually presents with pulmonary hypertension if symptomatic. Patients may have a characteristic **waterhammer pulse**. This is made more obvious by raising the patient's arm over their head while using your other hand to support the patient's elbow. You will feel a collapsing pulse beating against your fingers. It is described as *collapsing* as you feel a strong large volume beat that disappears quickly as the blood is regurgitated back through the aortic valve. In such a case, expect a **wide pulse pressure** and a thrusting apex beat. The **early diastolic murmur** of AR is heard loudest at the left sternal edge with the patient sitting forward in ***expiration*** (as it is a left-sided murmur). In addition to this, there may be a mid-diastolic **Austin Flint murmur** produced by the vibration of the anterior cusp of the mitral valve as it is pummeled by jets of blood from both the left atrium and aorta.

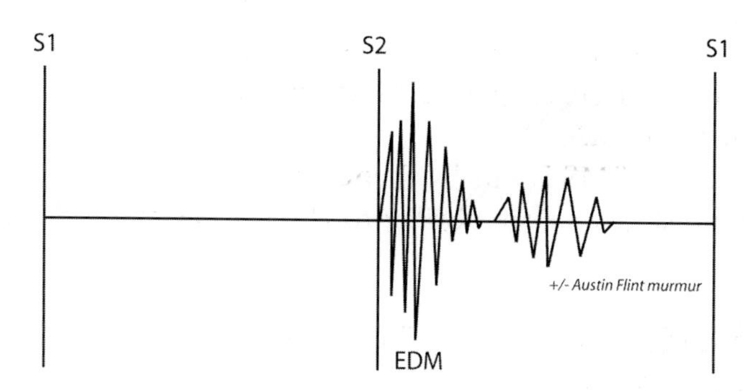

Figure 2.5 Aortic regurgitation

Aortic regurgitation is associated with over 30 eponymous signs; you don't need to know all of them but it's quite useful to remember a few:

- **Quincke's**: pulsating nail bed (get a senior to show you where to look so you know to look in the right place; or run up a couple of flights of stairs and see it in your own nail beds)
- **deMusset's**: head nodding
- **Corrigan's**: visible carotid pulsation
- **Duroziez's**: systolic and diastolic femoral murmurs
- **Traube's**: pistol shot femoral artery sounds

Again, look for features of cardiac failure and infective endocarditis.

The causes of AR can be divided into congenital and acquired. Acquired causes are:

- *Infective*: rheumatic? syphilitic?
- Inflammatory/Connective tissue diseases: Marfan's syndrome, ankylosing spondylitis, rheumatoid arthritis, systemic lupus erythematosus
- Traumatic

The investigations for this patient include:

- **ECG**: look for left ventricular hypertrophy (LVH)
- **Chest radiograph**: cardiomegaly

- **Echocardiography**: assess severity, left ventricular function, dimension, and cause
- **Catheterisation**

Management:

- *Surgical*: repair or replacement ideally before left ventricular dysfunction

2.4 Valve Replacement

Valves can generally be classified into mechanical and non-mechanical valves. The choice of valve depends on a number of factors including the age of the patient, risks of co-morbidities, and compliance to medication (for example, warfarin).

In some cases it may be appropriate to *consider a joint coronary artery bypass graft (CABG)/valve procedure* if the patient has concomitant coronary artery disease. Cardio-pulmonary bypass is necessary for all mitral valve repairs in order to create a bloodless field in which to operate.

Non-mechanical/bioprosthetic valves are commonly porcine or cadaveric. They last 10–15 years and are therefore generally reserved for the older patient. Look for a midline sternotomy scar or lateral thoracotomy scar for evidence of this. These valves produce normal heart sounds, although a flow murmur can sometimes be heard.

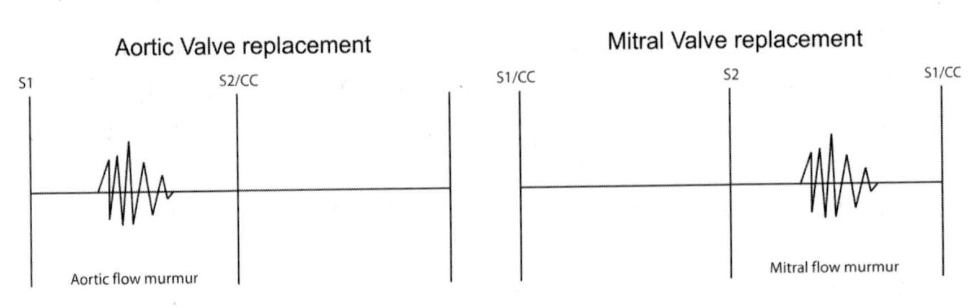

Figure 2.6 Comparing atrial valve and mitral valve replacement

Mechanical valves can be

- Ball and cage (Starr-Edwards)
- Tilting disc (Bjork-Shiley)
- Double tilting half-discs (St. Jude)

The default valve type is a metal valve. They last up to and beyond 20 years but require lifelong anticoagulation with warfarin.

When examining these patients, the closing of mechanical valves can be loud and sometimes heard from the end of the bed. This would correspond with S1 in a mitral valve replacement and S2 in an aortic replacement. (Some valves make a sound on opening, too.) A diastolic flow murmur is common across the mitral valve and likewise a systolic murmur across the aortic one.

If a patient has had a valve replacement, make note of whether the patient has any signs of a failing/leaking valve. In mitral valve replacement, this may present with signs consistent with mitral regurgitation — thus listen for a pansystolic murmur. In a leaking aortic valve, there may be an early diastolic murmur of aortic regurgitation.

The other complications of valve replacement include:

- **haemolysis**
- **bleeding (patients on warfarin therapy)**
- **thromboembolism**
- **infection → infective endocarditis**

The above valvular conditions are probably the commonest ones you will find on the wards. Bear in mind a patient may also present with a mixed picture of stenosis and regurgitation or mixed aortic and mitral disease. In these patients, one condition may predominate. Don't forget to always check the blood pressure and temperature chart and note what drugs he/she is taking.

The rarer conditions you may also come across include:

- Ventricular Septal Defect (VSD)
- Atrial Septal Defect (ASD)

- Patent Ductus Arteriosus (PDA)
- Coarctation of the aorta

2.5 Other Common Murmurs

2.5.1 *Ventricular septal defect (VSD)*

Ventricular septal defect is a differential for mitral regurgitation as it produces a **pansystolic murmur**. Keep this condition in mind if the patient is young. In clinical practice, watch out for this in anyone who has had a recent myocardial infarction (although the consequences are catastrophic and are unlikely to be conducive to the exam environment). The murmur tends to be localised to the left sternal edge with ***no radiation***. Look for signs of pulmonary hypertension, that is, loud P2, and RV heave and look for other associated signs, that is, aortic regurgitation, patent ductus arteriosus, tetralogy of Fallot, overriding aorta and coarctation. It is usually a congenital condition or can be acquired. The management of this patient depends on the size of the lesion. Small lesions tend to close spontaneously at a young age whereas closure is needed for haemodynamically significant lesions. Larger lesions run the risk of developing Eisenmenger's syndrome where there is a reversal of the left-right shunt.

> There is NO correlation between the size of a VSD lesion and the loudness of the murmur!

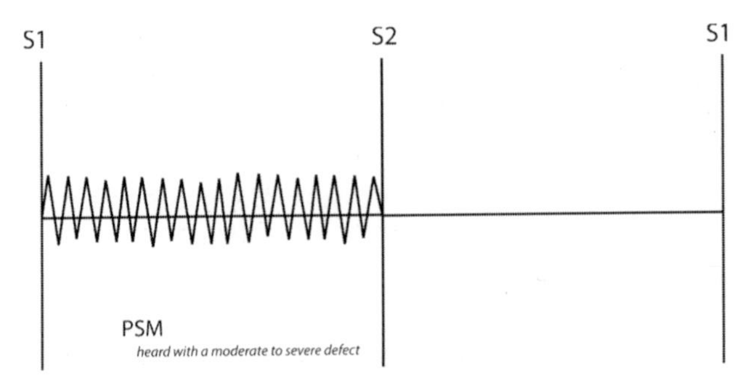

Figure 2.7 Ventricular septal defect

2.5.2 *Atrial septal defect (ASD)*

Atrial Septal Defect is another cause of an ejection systolic murmur — **ESM**. Consider this in younger patients. There may also be a diastolic component due to flow across the tricuspid valve. S2 is heard as a **fixed split heart sound** which means the time between the closure of the aortic valve and pulmonary valve is fixed and doesn't change with respiration. In normal patients, there is a physiological splitting of S2 during inspiration as a consequence of a decrease in intrathoracic pressure and an increase in systemic venous return to the right heart. The right ventricle takes slightly longer to eject this extra blood. The result is that pulmonary valve closure is delayed.

When examining a patient with an ASD, look for signs of cardiac failure and associated Down's syndrome facies. There are two types depending on the anatomical location: Primum and Secundum, of which Secundum is by far commoner. The complications of an ASD can be remembered by the acronym **PACE** — **P**aradoxical embolus, **atrial** arrhythmias, **C**ongestive cardiac failure and **E**ndocarditis. A Secundum septal defect can be repaired with a percutaneous umbrella device in many cases. Some cases, and most Primum cases, can only be dealt with by surgery.

A *paradoxical embolus* occurs as a clot from the venous system and passes through the septal defect into the arterial system.

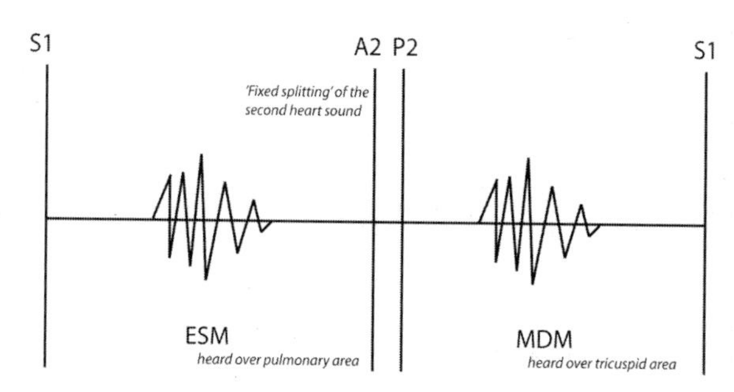

Figure 2.8 Atrial septal defect

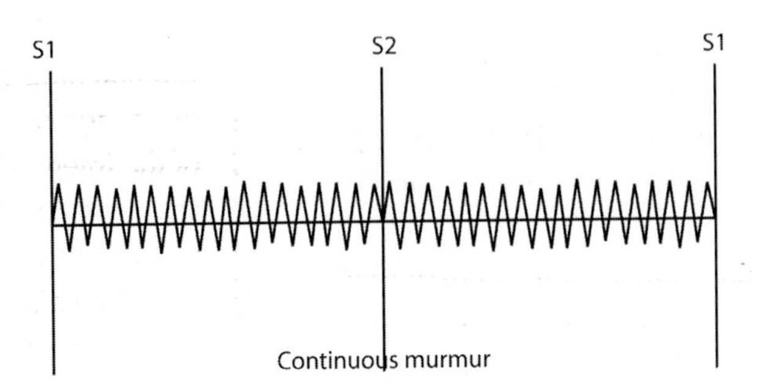

Figure 2.9 Patent ductus arteriosus

2.5.3 *Patent ductus arteriosus (PDA)*

The ductus arteriosus is the shunt connecting the pulmonary artery to the aortic arch that allows blood from the right ventricle to bypass the fetal lungs. A PDA occurs when this shunt fails to close following birth. It is more common in premature babies and infants with respiratory problems.

On examination, look out for the following:

- collapsing pulse
- prominent apical beat
- loud continuous 'machinery' murmur in second intercostals space

Palpable thrill

Management in the newborn involves indomethecin, a prostaglandin inhibitor to pharmacologically close the shunt if it is detected early, otherwise operational ligation and division is necessary with antibiotic cover.

2.5.4 *Coarctation of the aorta*

This is a congenital narrowing of the aorta usually distal to the left subclavian artery. The clinical signs associated with this condition are:

hypertension in right +/− left arm
prominent upper body pulses

Radiofemoral delay
heaving apex beat
continuous murmur radiating through
to the back (late presentation)

Rib notching occurs due to the hypertrophy of the intercostals arteries taking blood around the coarctation as collaterals.

ECG may show left ventricular hypertrophy and right bundle branch block. A chest radiograph may show rib notching and a double aortic knuckle. Management requires a balloon angioplasty, stenting and long-term anti-hypertensives.

2.6 Other Bedside Conditions

As a student on the wards, you will come across patients in all stages of their condition as well as in various stages of the hospital pathway. For some, it may be their first presentation of their disease, whereas others may have been admitted several times before for the same condition. Some patients will be awaiting investigations or even surgery. It is important to recognise some of the common scenarios as you may be in a situation where you may need to respond accordingly.

2.6.1 *Infective endocarditis (IE)*

It is already evident to you that patients with valvular disease are more susceptible to IE. Other risk factors include intravenous drug use, which predisposes patients to *staphylococcus aureus* vegetation on the *tricuspid valve* (this is the first valve the organism encounters when injected into the bloodstream), congenital heart disease, as well as the use of central venous catheters.

The features to look out for when examining a patient with suspected IE can be divided into the following systems:

Systemic features include: fever, night sweats, malaise, and weight loss

Hands: look for splinter haemorrhages, Osler nodes (**painful** red lesions on finger pulps), Janeway lesions (**painless** palmar nodules) and clubbing

Chest: **new murmur** or change in an existing one

Abdomen: splenomegaly, microscopic haematuria

Vasculitis

Embolic phenomenon: kidney, spleen, liver, and brain causing stroke

Janeway lesions are pathognomonic of IE due to a type III hypersensitivity reaction.

Although both are commonly mentioned by students, they are not common. Osler nodes occur in only 10–25% of patients.

It is best to stick to such a system as it makes it easier to remember and deliver on the spot. The investigations you should order when faced with such a patient include:

Urine dipstick: for blood

Bloods: full blood count (FBC), White cell count (WCC), Erythrocyte sedimentation rate (ESR)/C-reactive protein (CRP) and cultures

Transthoracic echo/transoesophageal echo: looking for vegetation

IE is diagnosed according to the **Duke criteria** and consists of either fulfillment of two major criteria, one major and three minor or all five minor criteria.

Table 2.2 Criteria for diagnosis of endocarditis

Major	Minor
+ Echo findings = vegetation + blood cultures	Fever + echo findings not meeting major criterion + blood cultures not meeting major criterion predisposition vascular/immunological signs

The commonest organisms to cause this condition are:

- *Streptococcus viridans*
- *Enterococcus*
- *Staphylococcus aureus* (particularly in intravenous drug users)

The management of such a patient will depend on blood culture sensitivities; however, the empirical treatment prior to gaining results from the lab will consist of a combination such as *benzylpenicillin* and *gentamicin* to cover gram-negative organisms.

Previously, antibiotic prophylaxis was routinely recommended for various interventional procedures for patients considered to be at high risk of infective endocarditis, that is, patients with valvular heart disease, structural congenital heart disease, valve replacement and previous infective endocarditis. However, recent research shows this is neither clinically, nor cost effective. **NICE guidelines 2008** do not recommend antibiotic prophylaxis to these high-risk patients undergoing dental procedures, procedures involving the upper and lower gastrointestinal tract, genitourinary tract, upper and lower respiratory tract.

2.6.2 *Rheumatic fever*

Students often get asked what this is as it is a typical screening question in history taking and a predisposing factor for valvular disease. Succinctly put, it is a childhood throat infection from Group A beta-haemolytic streptococcus that develops into a severe immune-mediated illness (often requiring hospitalisation for arthritis — hence the name) and then subsides, but which can cause valve disease some 10–20 years later.

The criterion for this condition is called the **Duckett Jones criteria** and the five major criteria can be remembered by the mnemonic '**CANES**':

1. **C**arditis — pancarditis (peri-, myo-, endocarditis/vasculitis)
2. **A**rthritis, migratory, polyarticular with fevers, Jaccoud's Arthropathy (swan-neck)

3. **N**odules, Subcutaneous — firm, usually over bony prominences or tendons
4. **E**rythema marginatum — evanescent pink rash, trunk and proximal extremities
5. **S**ydenham's Chorea — Abrupt and purposeless involuntary movements, usually of the hands and face

The management of this condition in the acute phase, now rare in the UK, consists of high dose aspirin and penicillin and prophylactic penicillin for five years.

2.6.3 *Patients on warfarin*

Ascertain the underlying diagnosis, which will give you an indication of the international normalised ratio (INR) you are trying to achieve. You may find patients on the wards on warfarin for various reasons including:

- deep vein thrombosis
- pulmonary embolism
- those with atrial fibrillation at risk of embolism
- mechanical heart valves

Drugs which interact with warfarin
liver enzyme inducers/inhibitors
analgesics
antibiotics
cardiovascular
endocrine
alcohol

If in doubt, check!

Condition	**Target** INR
Atrial Fibrillation	2–3
Dilated Cardiomyopathy	2–3
Prosthetic heart valve	**2.5–3.5**

INR is the international normalised ratio, which is a measure of the slowness of the extrinsic pathway of coagulation. The normal range is 0.8–1.2.

Induction

A typical starting regimen may be 10mg on the first and second days followed by 5mg on the third with measurement of the INR. The subsequent doses depend on the INR and are usually between 3 and 9 mg. The dose must be taken at the **same** time each day and the INR checked daily when starting treatment. Remember that the anti-coagulant effect of warfarin takes at least 48–72 hours to develop fully and the first INR is commonly measured 16 hours after administration (that is, if warfarin was administered at 6pm, the INR will be measured at 9am the next morning). Once an appropriate INR is determined, the INR can be measured at longer intervals.

Complications

The main complication of warfarin use is the risk of **haemorrhage** which is why meticulous measurement of INR is essential. It is sometimes necessary to omit the dose of warfarin such as in the event of a major bleed. Rarely, it may be necessary to give 1–10mg vitamin K (phytomenadione) by slow iv infusion, although this can make it very difficult to re-warfarinise the patient in the near future. Other agents used to reverse over-warfarinisation are prothrombin complex concentrate (factor II, VII, IX and X) and fresh frozen plasma.

In the event of surgery

In the event of surgery, there is a fine balance between the risk of bleeding and that of thromboembolism. Generally, warfarin needs to be stopped 3–5 days prior to surgery. In patients with metallic heart valves where the risk of thromboses is high, warfarin is converted to a low molecular weight heparin, or infusion pump of unfractionated heparin which is stopped 24–48 hours prior to the operation. The INR should be checked on admission. There are certain exceptions where warfarin does not need to be stopped, that is, for ophthalmic surgery and dental extractions. After the operation, patients can be restarted on warfarin on the evening of the same day.

In pregnancy

Warfarin is teratogenic and is contra-indicated in the first trimester of pregnancy (use heparin injections instead) and should be avoided if possible in later stages.

2.6.4 *Patients undergoing angiography*

You will come across both pre- and post-angiography patients on the wards. Prior to such a procedure, the patient would normally need pretreatment with both aspirin and heparin to thin the blood as well as the following investigations:

- blood tests including electrolytes, in particular to check renal function prior to contrast!
- ECG
- angiogram
- consent

During consent, the procedure itself, side effects, risks and complications should be explained to the patient. The complications can be divided into general and specific ones:

An *angiogram* is a real-time radiograph taken of the coronary vasculature. A catheter is introduced in either a femoral or radial artery and advanced around the aortic arch until it sits in the ostium of the coronary artery. Through the catheter, a dye is injected and real-time images can be taken of the moving blood in the vessels. Narrowed sections of the arteries can be visualised. (Refer to *Chapter 3 Investigations* for more information.)

Table 2.3 Complications of angiography

General	Specific
Bleeding	Restenosis
Infection	Dislodgement of a clot inducing a MI/stroke
Allergic reaction to anaesthetic	Death <5/1000

An *angioplasty* is the therapeutic manipulation of the narrowed stenosed coronary vessels. A balloon can be introduced via the catheter which can be inflated to widen a stenosed section of the artery. A stent can then be put in place to hold open the narrowed artery.

The angiogram is performed in a catheterisation lab and usually requires an overnight hospital stay. It lasts about 30 minutes and can be performed under local anaesthetic.

Back on the wards after the procedure, in some cases the arterial sheath is kept in for about 4 hours until the effects of the heparin have resolved. In other cases, the sheath is removed and a closure device applied. Patients are usually advised to lie flat for a couple of hours and ECG monitoring is maintained. However, an increase or new onset chest pain (especially with new ST or T wave changes) can signify abrupt occlusion of the vessel which may warrant immediate return to the catheterisation lab for re-opening.

Before discharging such patients, the following needs to be arranged:

- a follow-up appointment
- antiplatelet medicines
- advice on diet, lifestyle and driving.

2.6.5 *Patients who have had a coronary artery bypass graft*

To identify patients who have had a CABG in the past, in addition to a **median sternotomy scar**, also look for a possible saphenous vein harvest scar in the leg (the internal mammary artery is harvested without its own scar, via the median sternotomy) or a radial artery harvest scar. Bear in mind that the long saphenous vein is also used in a fem-pop bypass for peripheral artery disease. This will help you to differentiate those patients who have had a bypass and those who have had valvular surgery. Although you should keep in mind that they may have had both!

Chapter 3

Investigations

Investigations are an essential part of the patient-work up and are often asked about in undergraduate exams. When it comes to ordering investigations, the challenge lies not only in knowing which tests to request in order to confirm or exclude a diagnosis, but also the significance and interpretation of the results. In conjunction with the previous chapter on commonly encountered conditions, this chapter will give you an in-depth understanding of these everyday requests, ranging from 'blood tests' to angiograms and beyond.

3.1 Blood Tests

First line investigations are usually blood tests. These can be divided into **general** tests and blood tests **specific** to the diagnosis of certain cardiovascular conditions, namely *myocardial infarction* (*MI*) and *heart failure*. Also, given the large number of drugs used in cardiology, there is also a need to use blood tests for therapeutic monitoring of drug levels (that is, digoxin, warfarin and amiodarone).

3.1.1 *General blood tests*

All tests cost money and although it is easy to shout out the first test that pops into your head when asked, "What tests would you do on this patient?" the smart student would consider which tests are worth doing and more importantly, *why* they should be done.

However, if you consider what the likely diagnosis is (from history and examination) you can tailor your answers to properly justify the tests you are requesting.

Routine blood test and their significance in the patient with cardiovascular disease

- **Full blood count (FBC)**
  - *Haemoglobin*: Low haemoglobin known as anaemia is a cause of heart failure and breathlessness.
  - *White cell count (WCC)*: A raised WCC may occur in inflammation/infarction (for example, post-myocardial infarction). If prolonged pyrexia exists in conjunction with a new onset murmur, consider bacterial endocarditis (especially if the patient has a mechanical heart valve(s), a history of rheumatic fever or intravenous drug use [IVDU]).
  - *Platelet count*: Raised platelets, known as thrombocytosis, increase the likelihood of thrombosis. If low, consider heparin-induced thrombocytopenia (HIT) — see the *Heparin* section of Chapter 5 *Drugs* for more information.

- **Urea and Electrolytes (U&Es)**
  Urea and electrolytes are useful in assessing kidney function in a patient with cardiovascular disease for several reasons:
  - Chronic kidney disease is an independent risk factor for cardiovascular disease.
  - Kidney dysfunction may co-exist in patients with hypertension, diabetes, and peripheral arterial disease.
  - Kidney dysfunction may be a consequence of cardiovascular drugs, such as, diuretics and angiotensin converting enzyme (ACE) inhibitors.

  Although a raised urea and creatinine is indicative of kidney disease, the glomerular filtration rate is more useful at assessing the degree of renal impairment.

  Specific abnormalities include:
  - Low sodium — this may indicate fluid overload which can precipitate heart failure.
  - High or low potassium may induce arrhythmias.

  - Abnormalities in calcium, magnesium, and phosphate can also precipitate arrhythmias and should be corrected in the first instance.

Note: Low sodium and potassium may be secondary to diuretic treatment.

- **C Reactive Protein (CRP)** — CRP is raised in inflammation and infarction (for example, post-myocardial infarction). There is also emerging evidence to show that CRP may be a prognostic factor in vascular risk underlying the theory that atherosclerosis is an inflammatory process.
- **Clotting Profile** — Deranged clotting may be an indication of underlying hypercoagulopathy and can predispose patients to thromboembolism. Patients with atrial fibrillation or mechanical heart valves on warfarin require monitoring of their international normalised ratio (INR) (see Chapter 5 *Drugs*).
- **Lipid Profile** — The lipid profile includes triglycerides, total-cholesterol, high density lipoprotein (HDL) cholesterol and low density lipoprotein (LDL) cholesterol. It is recommended by the British Heart Society that all patients over 40 should have their cholesterol levels measured as part of a cardiovascular risk assessment in primary care. A fasting sample (after at least 12 hours of fasting) should be taken prior to lipid lowering treatment and the result used in conjunction with other risk factors including blood pressure, glucose and body weight to calculate a total risk.

  - The risk of cardiovascular disease increases with increasing concentrations of total cholesterol and LDL cholesterol. (See Chapter 5 *Drugs* section.)
  - HDLs transport cholesterol back to the liver and therefore levels of HDL are inversely proportional to cardiovascular risk.
  - Triglycerides are loosely associated with a risk of cardiovascular disease.

Remember, secondary causes of elevated lipids such as alcohol abuse, diabetes, renal disease and liver disease should be investigated before starting drug treatment.

Table 3.1 Definition of diabetes

	Fasting plasma glucose	Random plasma glucose test	Oral glucose tolerance test
Normal	<6 mmol/l		<7.8 mmol/l
Impaired glucose tolerance	>6 to <7 mmol/l		>7.8 mmol/l to <11.1 mmol/l
Diabetes	>7 mmol/l	>11.1 mmol/l	>11.1 mmol/l

- **Glucose** — High blood glucose is another independent risk factor in cardiovascular disease. It is associated with a twofold increase in cardiovascular risk in women and a threefold increase in the risk for men. Again, the British Heart Society recommends that all adults over 40 should have a random glucose measurement as part of a cardiovascular risk assessment in primary care.
  - If the non-fasting glucose is >6 mmol/l but <7 mmol/l, then repeat a fasting glucose (at least 8 hours fasting) on a different day.
  - The oral glucose tolerance test is performed when two fasting glucose readings taken on two different days is >7 mmol/l. Diabetes is confirmed if the glucose reading is >11.1 mmol/l after the oral glucose tolerance test.

3.1.2 *Specific tests*

Myocardial infarction (MI)

Myoglobin

- Low molecular weight haem protein binds O_2 in muscles.
- Present in all muscle cells including skeletal and cardiac muscle and released on damage so not specific to MI.
- Levels rise quickly post-MI (<4 hours) and return to normal after 8–12 hours.
- Normal myoglobin makes the diagnosis unlikely in the early stages.

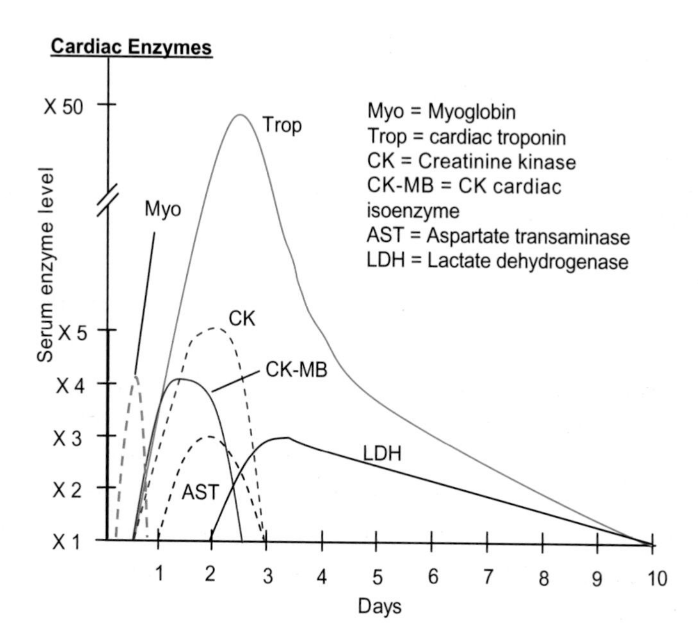

Figure 3.1 A graph showing the changes in cardiac enzyme levels with time post-chest pain

In the event of a myocardial infarction, death of cardiac myocytes results in the release of a number of cardiac proteins into the blood stream. There is a specific order and timing for the release of these proteins, and it is important to know these so that you know which tests would yield the most useful results depending on length of time from the onset of symptoms (Fig. 3.1). This is a popular topic for ward rounds and exams.

In order of time detectable after chest pain, the important ones are:

- Myoglobin
- **Creatinine kinase (CK)**
- **Troponin I or T**
- Aspartate aminotransferase (AST).

In clinical practice, CK and troponin are the main ones used for the diagnosis of acute myocardial infarction (see the Appendix for the criteria for diagnosis). CK and AST are enzymes. The other two are not, but sometimes the whole basket of proteins is loosely described as '**cardiac enzymes**'.

Creatinine kinase (CK)

This muscle enzyme has two subunits: Muscle (M) and Brain (B). The subunits combine to form three isoenzymes, CK-MM (in skeletal muscle), CK-BB (in the brain) and **CK-MB** (in cardiac muscle).

The cardiac muscle contains 30% CK-MB whereas skeletal muscle contains less than 3% CK-MB (>97% CK-MM) and so damage to cardiac muscle releases a larger proportion of CK-MB compared to CK-MM. The immunoassay assesses the percentage of total CK made up by CK-MB: <3% is normal; >5% is diagnostic of an MI. Levels rise 6–10 hours post-chest pain and peak at 12–24 hours. The levels normalise by 48–72 hours but will **rise again if there is a re-infarct**. CK-MB used to be the gold standard test for detecting MI but has now been superseded by troponins.

Troponins

These are part of the complex regulating actin-myosin complexes in all muscle cells. However, Troponin isoforms **I** (Inhibitory troponin) and **T** (troponin-Tropomysin) are specific for cardiac myocytes. Of the two types of troponins commonly in use, the I isoform is said to be slightly more specific than the T isoform, however both are considered **gold standards** for detecting an acute MI.

Almost all healthy normal people have extremely low levels of troponin but levels are very **sensitive and specific** to even minor cardiac damage. Yet it is important to measure plasma levels at the appropriate time — this is best measured from **12 hours** after the onset of chest pain (hence it is imperative that you establish **when** the pain started). Unlike CK, troponin levels stay high for **7–10 days** post-MI and so are useful for retrospective diagnosis of silent MI but are less useful for detecting re-infarction within a few days.

Table 3.2 Other causes of a raised troponin

Cardiac	Non-cardiac
Myocarditis	Renal failure
Cardiomyopathy	Pulmonary embolism
Heart failure	Sepsis and septic shock
Post-angiogram +/– angioplasty	Stroke
Cardiac surgery	Endurance exercise (marathon runners!)

A favourite question on ward rounds, in cath-labs and the Emergency Department is, "What are the 'other' causes of a raised troponin?" Answering this with confidence will not only impress your seniors, but will also prevent unnecessary angst in that elderly gentleman with a borderline raised troponin level on the renal unit.

To Impress!

Treatment options in the case of a suspected myocardial infarction should not be dependent on the results of troponins or CK. The diagnosis should be made by symptoms and ECG findings. If there is doubt as to the diagnosis, the ideal treatment is emergency coronary angiography and angioplasty if required.

Lastly, there are two other enzymes to mention — **lactate dehydrogenase** (LDH) and transaminase **aspartate** (AST). Historically, they were valuable because they remained elevated for many days, but with the advent of troponin testing, they are almost obsolete.

LDH

- Two of five isoenzymes are specific for cardiac myocytes.
- LD1 (hydroxybutyrate dehydrogenase [HBD]) and LD2.
- In myocardial infarction, there is a rise of LD1 relative to LD2.
- Levels rise and remain high for 7–10 days.
- Useful if no CK is done in the first 24 hours (retrospective diagnosis).
- Largely obsolete in most hospitals.

AST

- Released by damaged cardiac myocytes.
- Also found in hepatocytes.
- Not specific for MI.
- Levels rise 6–10 hours after pain, peak at 12–24 hours and normalise after 72 hours.

Heart failure

There are two main neurohormonal peptides secreted by the heart. They are:

- **A** — atrial Natriuretic peptide (ANP)
- **B** — brain (B-type) Natriuretic peptide (BNP).

Atrial natriuretic peptide (ANP)

ANP is an amino acid released by the atria of the heart in response to high blood pressure. It has a role in the homeostasis of water, sodium, potassium and adipose tissue.

Brain natriuretic peptide (BNP)

BNP is another amino acid released from the ventricles of the heart in response to excessive myocyte stretching. Thus it is used as both a **diagnostic and prognostic marker in patients with left ventricular failure** with over 90% and 60% sensitivity and specificity respectively.

Limitations of BNP

The disadvantage is that it does not give a useful idea as to the cause of the abnormality, be it myocardial infarction, valvular disease or other cardiomyopathy. Echocardiography is required to achieve this. Therefore, in hospital practice, BNP is often not used for the diagnosis of heart failure because echocardiography is more readily available.

In the community, however, far from an echocardiogram, even an imperfect sensitivity and specificity is attractive. BNP is also useful in the screening of low-risk individuals for possible heart failure, and also for tracking the progress of patients with heart failure, for example in research studies.

3.2 Electrocardiography (ECG)

Reading, reporting and interpreting ECGs is an essential tool for all clinicians. From the care-of-elderly ward through to the surgical ward and beyond, this is a skill to be mastered! How? Practice, practice, practice!

At first glance the ECG may seem daunting and overwhelming. However, having a systematic approach will help you to become competent at this task. Let us begin by reviewing the electrical system of the heart.

3.2.1 *Cardiac conduction pathway explained — The 3-step approach*

Step 1

Impulses are generated at the sinoatrial node (SAN) — they depolarise the atria resulting in the **P wave** (atrial depolarisation). Both the right and left atria contract simultaneously emptying blood out of the atria into the ventricles.

Step 2

These impulses are then propagated to the ventricles passing firstly through the AV node, and then the His bundle, via the Bundle Branches enroute to the apex of the heart. **PR interval** represents AV nodal delay (to allow ventricular filling).

Step 3

From the apex, the Purkinje fibres then carry the impulse to the myocytes around the heart (epicardium) and those within (endocardium)

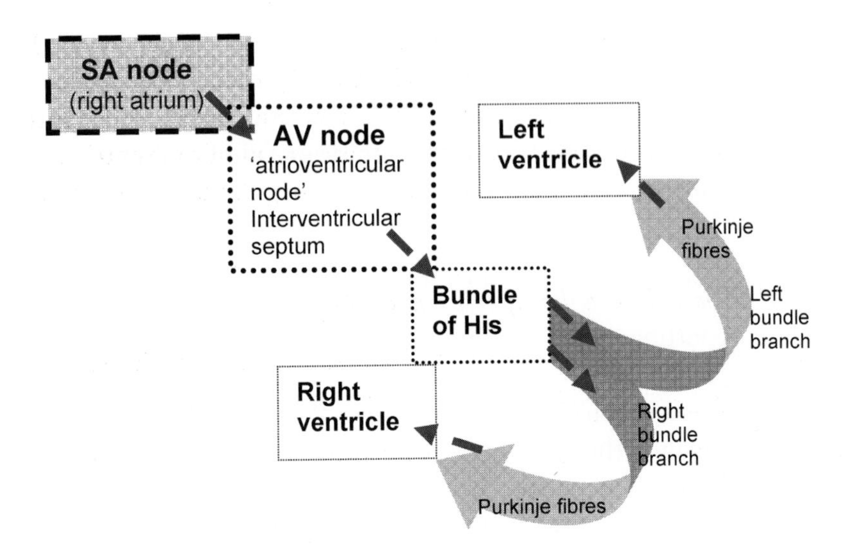

Figure 3.2 The electrical conduction system of the heart: conduction pathway (diagram above) and resultant ECG (diagram below)

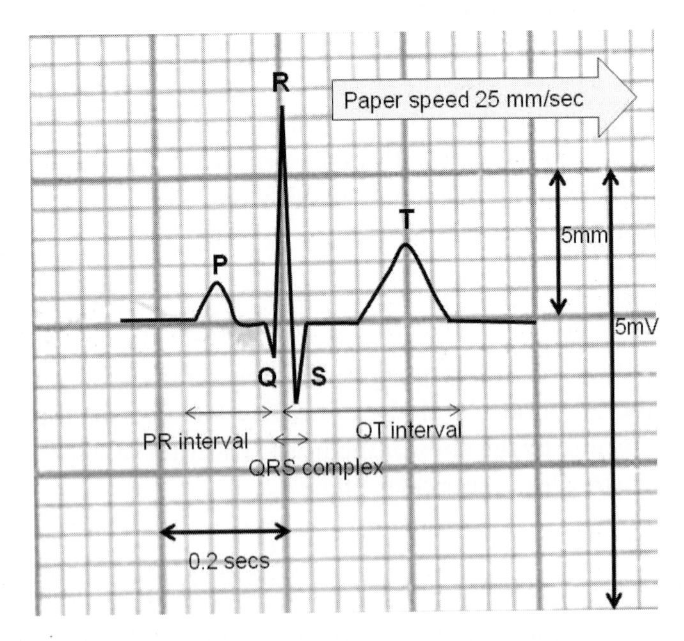

Figure 3.3 Foundations of the ECG waves

resulting in simultaneous contraction of the cells of the ventricles (depolarisation of the ventricles → **QRS complex**), squeezing blood out into the great vessels (pulmonary artery and aorta). The ventricles then relax corresponding to the repolarisation of the ventricles → **T wave**. The **ST segment** represents the beginning of ventricular repolarisation.

3.2.2 *When should I request an ECG?*

Remember that there are cardiac and non-cardiac reasons for requesting an ECG. They include:

Common cardiac symptoms — chest pain, palpitations, syncope

Cardiac indications

- Ischaemia/infarction
- Acute coronary syndrome
- Screening tool for cardiac ischaemia — exercise tolerance test (ETT)
- Arrhythmia/conduction abnormalities
- Tachy- and bradyarrhythmias
- Heart block/bundle branch blocks
- Electrolyte abnormalities:
  - hypo/hyperkalaemia,
  - hypo/hypercalcaemia
- Cardiac disease:
  - Hypertension
  - Valvulopathy, that is, mitral stenosis may result in atrial fibrillation (AF)
  - Cardiomyopathy
- Suspected drug overdose — i.e. digoxin

Non-cardiac indications

- Pulmonary embolism
- Hypothermia
- Pre-operative assessment

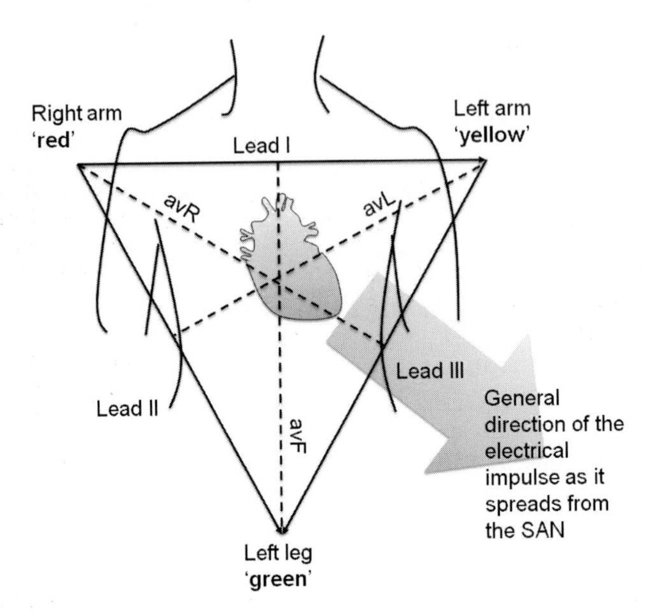

Figure 3.4 Orientation of chest and limb leads

3.2.3 *Where do I place the ECG leads?*

The mnemonic '**R**ide **y**our **g**reen **b**ike' is often used as a reminder for placing the limb leads in the appropriate places. **R**ed lead (lead I) is place unto the **r**ight arm, **y**ellow lead (lead II) to **l**eft arm, **g**reen lead (lead III) to left leg (it may also help to remember that 'green' is for 'grass' so green lead to leg — left leg!). The **b**lack lead is the reference lead — it is seldom used in practice.

Augmented leads

These are not actual leads placed on the patient, but are formed as vectors from the existing limb leads. aVR (towards Right arm), aVL (towards Left arm), and aVF (towards Left leg).

Limb leads

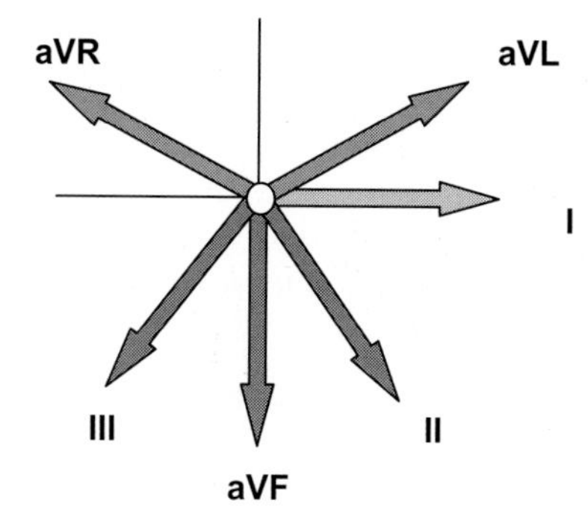

Anterior leads V_{1-6} represents the anterior wall of the heart (the frontal wall of the left ventricle).

Lateral leads I, aVL, V_5 & V_6 represent the lateral wall of the heart (lateral wall of the left ventricle).

Inferior leads II, III & **aVF** reflect the inferior wall of the heart (apex of left ventricle).

Chest leads

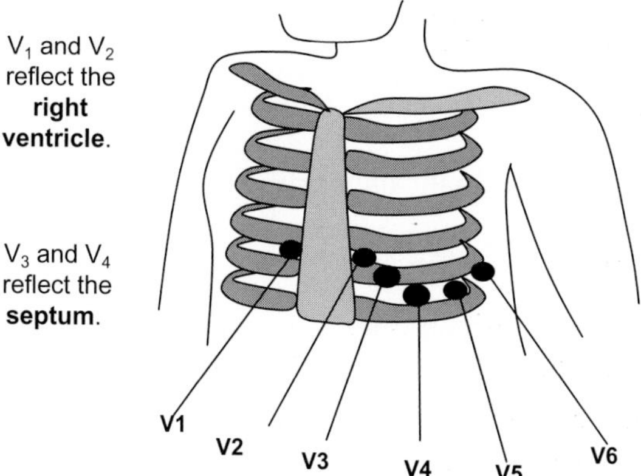

V_5 and V_6 reflect the **lateral** and **anterior** wall of the **left ventricle**.

Figure 3.5 Interpretation of chest and limb leads

Must know ECG tips:

- Check that the machine is calibrated to run at a speed of 25 mm/second.
- 1 mV = 10 mm (or 1 cm = two large squares) so at a standard signal of 1 mV, the stylus moves upwards to a height of 1cm.

Note: The height of the complexes may indicate pathology, such as, ventricular hypertrophy (if very tall) or pericardial effusion (if very short).

Attachment of the chest (V leads) overlies the fourth and fifth rib spaces as shown above.

3.2.4 *What does this ECG show?*

If you have not already encountered this question — then you need to spend more time on the wards! Do not panic! Always begin with the basics.

'*This is the ECG of* [insert patient name] *taken on the* [insert date] *at* [insert time]'.

Quickly check the paper speed and calibration to ensure that it is standard (25 mm/sec; 1 cm = 1 mV) (see above). Then report the following:

1. **Rhythm**
2. **Rate**
3. **Cardiac axis**

Having established these, systematically analyse the complex in each lead.

4. **P waves**
5. **PR intervals**
6. **QRS complexes**
7. **ST segment**
8. **T waves**
9. **Localise the underlying pathology**
10. **Summarise your findings**

3.2.5 *Rhythm*

The rhythm is either 'sinus' or 'non-sinus', such as, atrial fibrillation (see *Chapter 4 Commonly Encountered Patients*). Sinus rhythm occurs when a P wave precedes every QRS complex (see below), indicating that atrial depolarisation is initiated at the sinoatrial node. If the rhythm is irregular, and there are no obvious P waves, then atrial fibrillation is likely.

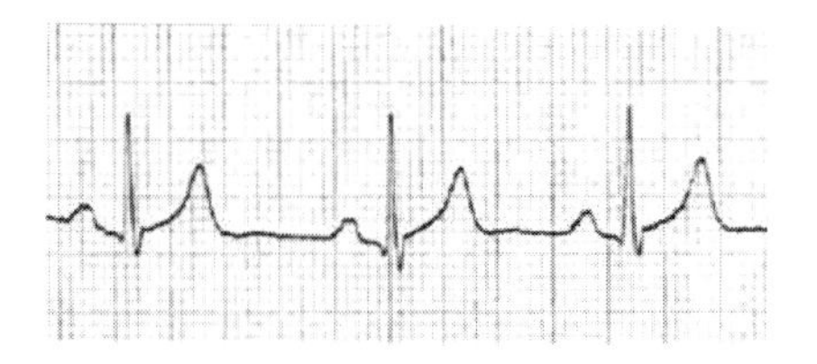

Figure 3.6 Sinus rhythm

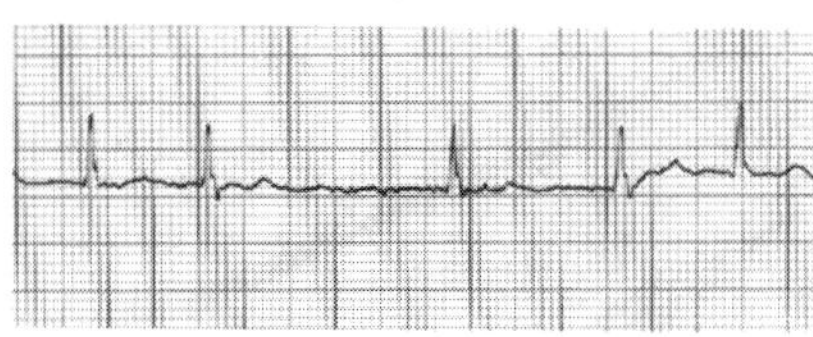

Figure 3.7 Atrial fibrillation

3.2.6 *Rate*

Normal heart rate is ~70 bpm (rate set by depolarisation at the sinoatrial node). Seventy to one hundred bpm is within the acceptable range.

- **Bradycardia HR ≤ 60 bpm**
- **Tachycardia HR ≥ 100 bpm**.

For more information on causes and management of brady- and tachyarrhythmias see (*Chapter 4 on Arrhythmias*).

How to calculate the heart rate

Each small square on the ECG rhythm strip is **0.04 seconds** long and each large square (consisting of five smaller ones), represents **0.20 seconds**. Therefore, when looking at an ECG, you can easily estimate the rate by looking at the number of large squares between the peak of the QRS complexes (R to R interval). In the example below there are three large squares between the R waves, thus the heart rate is 300/3 = 100 beats per minute.

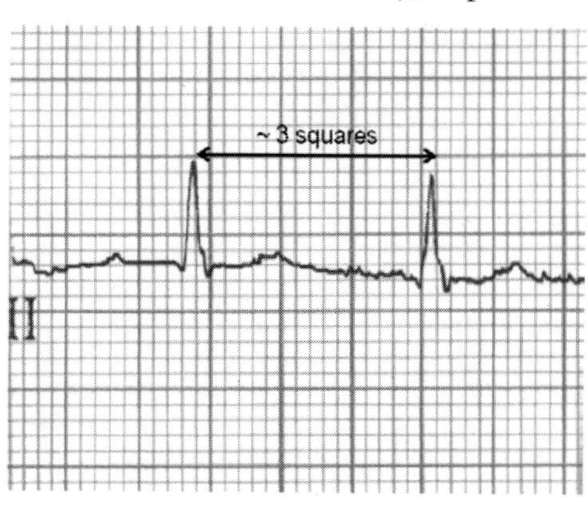

Figure 3.8 R-R interval

Table 3.3 Calculating heart rate

Number of squares between R waves	Beats per minute
1	300
2 (300 divided by 2)	150
3 (300 divided by 3)	100
4 (300 divided by 4)	75 etc.

3.2.7 *Cardiac axis*

Students can find determination of the cardiac axis a real challenge. If you do, you are not alone! The cardiac axis is the average direction of spread of the depolarisation across the ventricle. **Normal range is between –30° and +90°**.

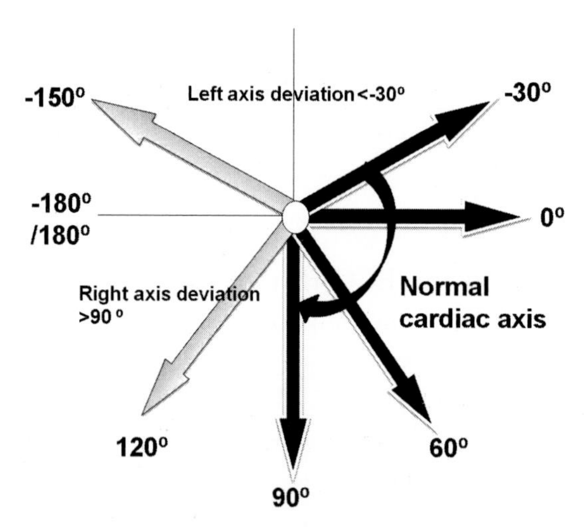

Figure 3.9 Cardiac axis wheel

To determine this, let's look at the deflection of the QRS complex. Normally the depolarisation spreads *towards* the direction of leads II, III, and aVF thus in these leads, the QRS deflection is positive (that is, an upwards peak).

However in **L**eft **A**xis **D**eviation (**LAD** < **–30°**), the depolarisations are predominantly ***away from leads II***, thus the QRS deflection is negative (downwards peak/prominent 'Q' in leads II, III, and aVF).

In **R**ight **A**xis **D**eviation (**RAD** > **+90°**) it is predominantly ***away from lead I*** (negative QRS deflection in lead I).

In left ventricular hypertrophy (LVH), the increase LV bulk causes a conduction defect. The cardiac axis is < –30° (**LAD**), that is, away from lead II, **QRS lead II is negative → downward peak** (see Table 3.4).

Thus in right ventricular hypertrophy (RVH), the cardiac axis is >+90° (**RAD**), that is, **QRS lead I is negative** and QRS lead III positive (see Table 3.4).

Table 3.4 Direction of the cardiac axis

	Normal axis	**L**eft **A**xis **D**eviation	**R**ight **A**xis **D**eviation
Lead I	+ QRS	**+ QRS**	**– QRS**
Lead II	+ QRS	– QRS	+ QRS
Lead III/aVF	+ QRS	**– QRS**	**+ QRS**

3.2.8 *P wave*

Usually uniform, dome-shaped.

P wave represents atrial depolarisation from the sinoatrial node across both the right, and left atrium.

The **absence** of P wave before each QRS complex suggests dys-synchronous atrial activity, that is, atrial fibrillation.

Abnormal P waves:

- **Bifid P wave** (*'p mitrale'*) as in **Left Atrial Hypertrophy**
  Causes: Mitral/aortic stenosis/regurgitation, cardiomyopathy
  Tip: Best seen in lead II

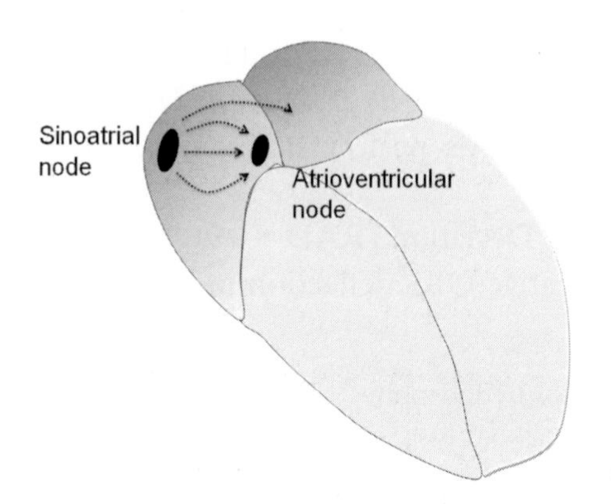

Figure 3.10 Atrial depolarisation

- **Peaked P wave** suggest **Right Atrial Hypertrophy** ∧
  Causes: Tricuspid stenosis, cor pulmonale, pulmonary hypertension
  Tip: Best seen in leads I–III

3.2.9 *PR interval*

Normally 120–200 ms (three to five small squares).
Abnormal PR interval:

- **First degree heart block** — prolong PR interval >200 ms (five small squares), but each P wave is followed by a QRS complex.
- **Second degree heart block**
  In this cardiac conduction defect, there is failure of some P waves being conducted to the ventricle to generate a QRS complex. Consequently some P waves are not followed by a QRS complex.

There are two types of second degree heart block:

i) Mobitz type I (known as 'Wenckebach phenomenon'), and
ii) Mobitz type II.

Mobitz type 1 (Wenckebach first described this in humans in 1898!)
There is progressive prolongation of the PR interval, until a P wave is

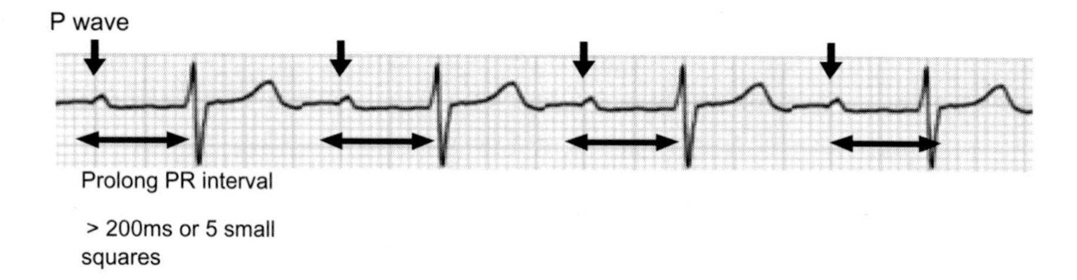

Figure 3.11 First degree heart block

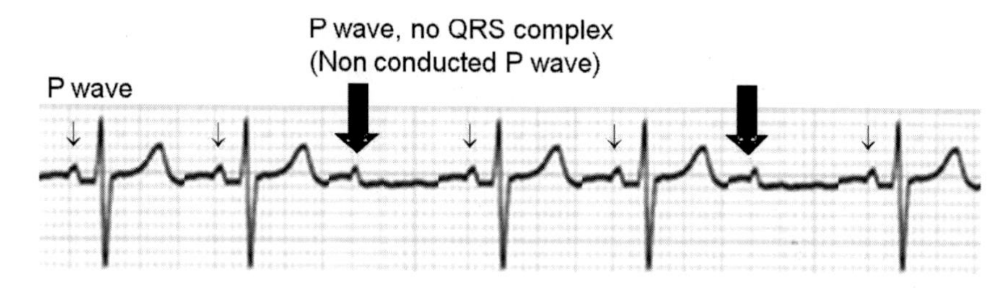

Figure 3.12a Mobitz type II

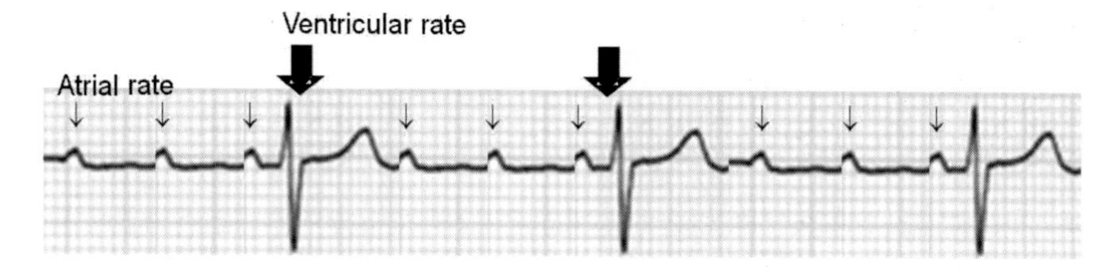

Figure 3.12b Third degree heart block

'blocked' (that is, not conducted to the ventricle, hence the P wave is not followed by a QRS complex).

Mobitz type II Intermittent episodes of non-conducted 'blocked' P waves, associated with a **constant PR interval**.

- **Third degree heart block**
  The atria and ventricles are contrating independently of one another resulting in independent atrial and ventricular rates. Atrial

activity is not conducted to the ventricles hence the atrial rate is faster than the ventricular rate. The emerging QRS complex results from an abnormal depolarising focus in the ventricle (escape rhythm, hence the slow rate ~30 per minute).

3.2.10 *QRS complex*

Usually upward deflection (dominant R wave in limb leads), with R wave becoming more prominent from V1 to V6 (known as **'R wave progression'** — poor R wave progression may be indicative of an anterior infarct/left bundle branch block (LBBB), left/right ventricular hypertrophy (L/R VH) and WPW — Wolff-Parkinson-White.

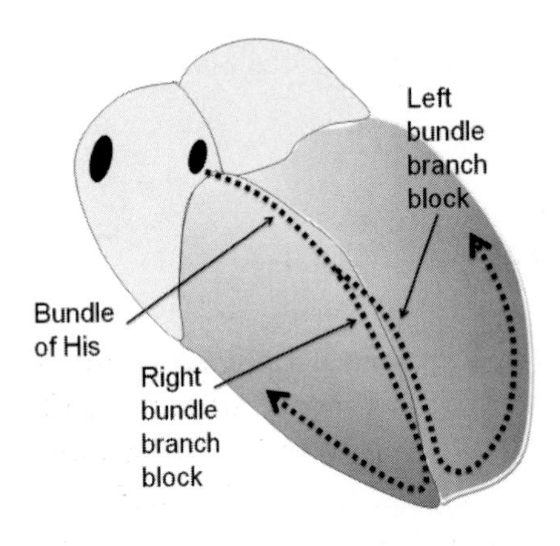

Figure 3.13 Ventricular depolarization Duration: 80–120 ms (2–3 small squares).

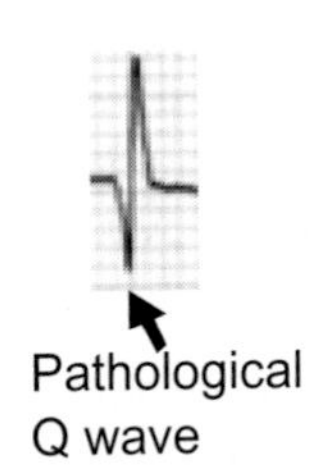

Figure 3.14 Pathological Q wave

Abnormalities in QRS complex:

- **Pathological Q wave:** >0.04 seconds in width and >2mm (two small squares in depth) or > one third of the R wave height.
- **Axis deviations** (see above)
  - Left **A**xis **D**uration (axis < −30°) — causes: Left bundle branch block, left ventricular hypertrophy, Inferior wall MI.

- ○ **R**ight **A**xis **D**eviation (axis > –90°) — causes: Right ventricular hypertrophy, dextrocardia (heart +/– other organs on the right side of the body instead of the left).

- **Left Ventricular Hypertrophy (LVH)** — tall R waves in the left ventricular leads and deep S waves in the right ventricular leads. **Note:** Voltage Criteria **SV_1 + RV_6 > 35 mm** (deep S wave in V1 added to tall R wave in V5/V6 is >7 large squares).
Causes: Hypertension, Aortic stenosis, and Cardiomyopathy.
- **Right Ventricular Hypertrophy** — Right axis deviation or R wave (>S wave in V1 or > 7 mm).
Causes: Pulmonary stenosis and pulmonary hypertension.

Wide QRS complexes

Always consider bundle branch block (**BBB**).

There are two types of bundle branch block:

i) Left bundle branch block — LBBB, and
ii) Right bundle branch block — RBBB.

The mnemonic **'WiLLiaM MaRRoW'** refers to the QRS complex pattern in BBB. A 'W-pattern' is seen in V1 with an 'M-pattern' in V6 in Left BBB. In Right BBB, an 'M-pattern' is seen in V1 (known formally as an 'RSR' wave) with a 'W-pattern' in V6. Refer to accompanying examples of LBBB and RBB on ECG (see the Appendix).

***Note*: An ECG in a patient with suspected myocardial infarction in the presence of BBB is very difficult to interpret!**

3.2.11 *ST segment*

Although usually flat (isoelectric), it may also be 1 mm above or below the baseline.

Abnormal ST segment:

- Four causes of **ST segments** elevation are:
  - i) **Myocardial infarction** (acute ST Elevation Myocardial Infarction — STEMI). 1–2 mm elevation in ≥2 leads from the same region of the heart (contiguous leads — see 'Anatomical localisation of myocardial infarction' below).
  - ii) Acute Pericarditis — widespread 'saddle-shaped' ST elevation in all leads except V1 +/– PR depression in leads II and V6 and PR elevation in aVR.
  - iii) Left ventricular aneurysm — always consider in patients with persistent ST elevation post-myocardial infarction.
  - iv) High take-off.

- Four causes of **ST segments depression** are:
  - i) **Myocardial ischaemia**, that is, Non-ST-Elevation MI (NSTEMI).
  - ii) **Digoxin effect** — check drug history and Digoxin level.
  - iii) **Acute posterior MI** — R wave and ST depression in V1–V3.
  - iv) **Pulmonary Embolus** — S1Q3T3 (prominent S wave in lead 1 with deep Q wave and T wave inversion in lead III — it is uncommon. Sinus tachycardia and atrial fibrillation are commoner ECG features in pulmonary embolus.

3.2.12 *T wave*

Normally upward deflection in leads I, II, and V3–V6.

Abnormal T wave

T wave inversion
Associated with myocardial ischaemia (regional ST depression is indicative of **Acute Coronary Syndromes** — Non-ST-Elevation-MI [NSTEMI]).

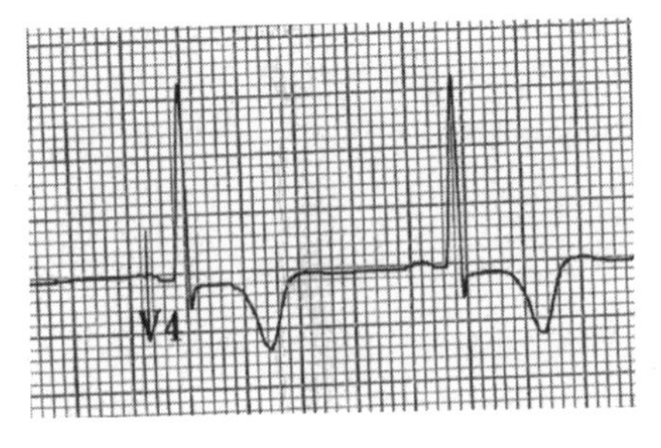

Figure 3.15 T wave inversion

- **Tall T waves**
  Hyperkalaemia — tall, 'tented' (peaked)
  T waves with flat P waves. Morphology changes with increasing levels of potassium.
- **Flat T waves**
  Hypokalaemia — flattening of T wave, ST depression, U waves (downward deflection immediately after T wave).

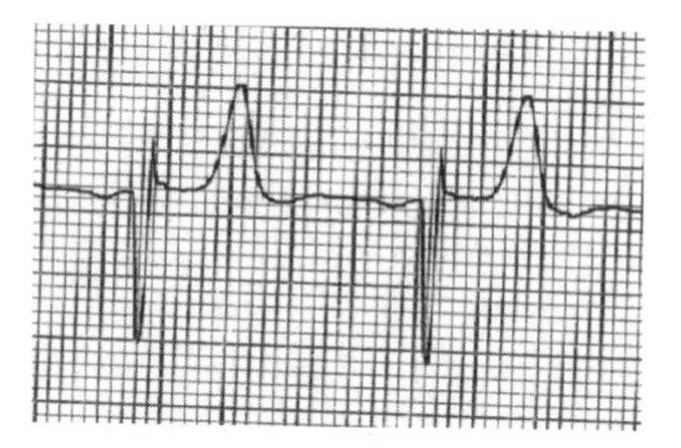

Figure 3.16 Tall T waves

3.2.13 *QT interval*

Normal QT interval is 300–460 ms.

Abnormal QT interval

Prolonged QT interval — 'long QT'. QT interval >460 ms. Causes include ***CDE:***

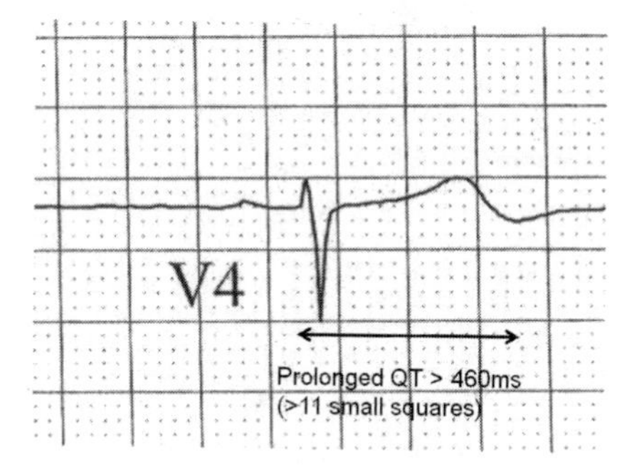

Figure 3.17 Long QT

- **C**ongenital long QT syndromes, that is, Romano Ward syndrome* or Lange Nielsen**.
- **D**rugs — especially anti-arrhythmics.
  - Mnemonic '***SAD Qupid***' — **S**otalol **A**miodarone **D**isopyramide, **Qui**nidine, **P**rocainam**id**e), Tricyclic anti-depressants, anti-psychotics.
- **E**lectrolyte abnormalities, that is, hypokalaemia,
- Hypomagnesaemia and hypocalcaemia.

---

*Romano Ward syndrome — Long QT and congenital deafness, autosomal dominant inheritance.

** Lange Nielsen — Long QT syndrome, autosomal recessive inheritance.

3.3 Anatomical Localisation of Myocardial Infarction

Now that you have understood how to read an ECG from earlier in this chapter, let us put this into practice by interpreting ECGs in the context of an acute MI. The challenge is to convert information in a 2D form, that is, the printed ECG in front of you, into where the heart attack is in the 3D structure of the patient's heart.

Firstly, a brief reminder of the arteries in the heart and the regions they supply. The right coronary artery (RCA) is in green, the left main stem (LMS) in blue, the left anterior descending artery (LAD) in pink and the circumflex in yellow. The colours of the myocardium in this picture reflect the origin of the blood supply to this region (see Fig. 3.18).

Acute myocardial infarction is represented on ECG in its classic form as elevation in the ST segment. In order to understand where on the heart the infarction is taking place, we first need to relate the leads on the 12 lead ECG to the anatomical position of the heart. Figure 3.19 below hows the direction of the limb and chest leads superimposed onto the heart as it would sit in the thorax.

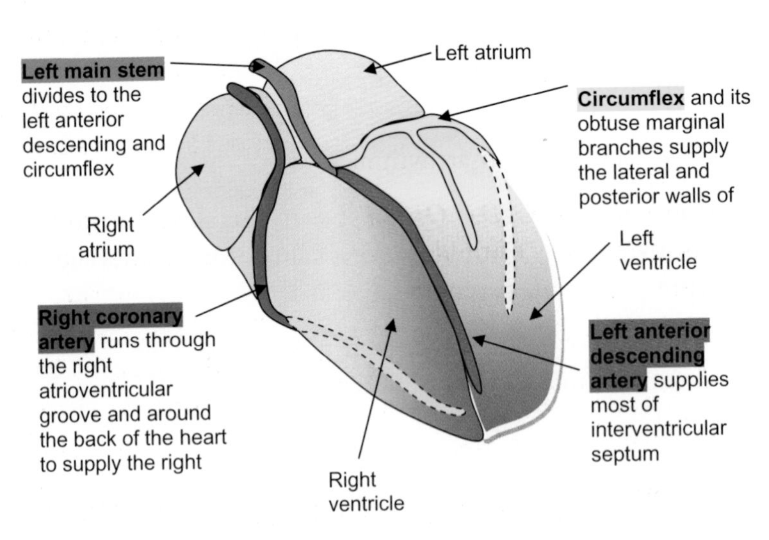

Figure 3.18 Diagram of coronary vasculature

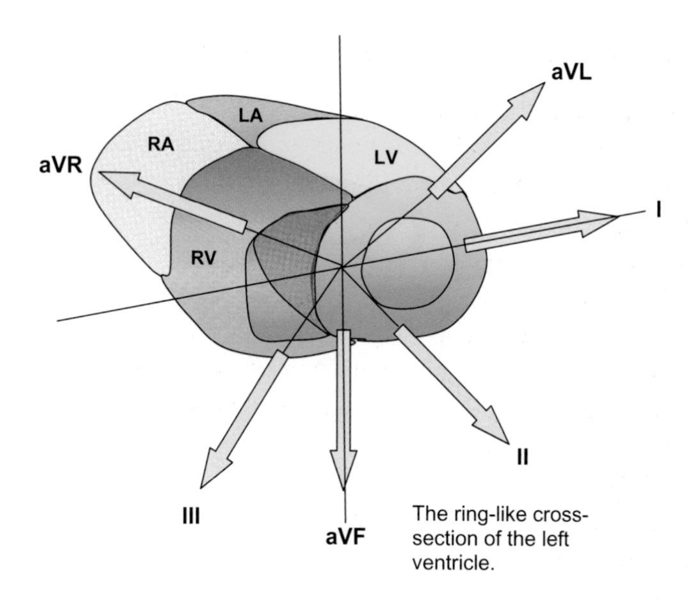

Figure 3.19 Localisation of limb leads

From the diagram you can see that leads I and aVL represent the overall conduction towards the left (lateral) wall of the left ventricle. Similarly, leads aVR represent the electrical conduction towards the right side of the heart and Leads II, III and aVF represent conduction to the inferior aspect of the heart (see Fig. 3.2).

So from the figure, should there be ST changes in leads I and aVL, this would be suggestive of infarction in the **lateral wall of the left ventricle**.

How can the chest leads help you at this stage? Figure 3.20 shows the chest leads and which areas of the heart they represent. V1 looks at the direction of conduction towards the right side of the heart predominantly supplied by the RCA. V2–4 reflects the anterior and septal wall the heart supplied predominantly by the LAD. V5–6 reflects the left lateral wall of the ventricle. Therefore, in a lateral infarction, we may also expect some ST elevation in leads V5–V6.

In our example above, ST elevation in leads I, aVL, V5–6 represent damage to the lateral ventricle of the heart. Correspondingly, on

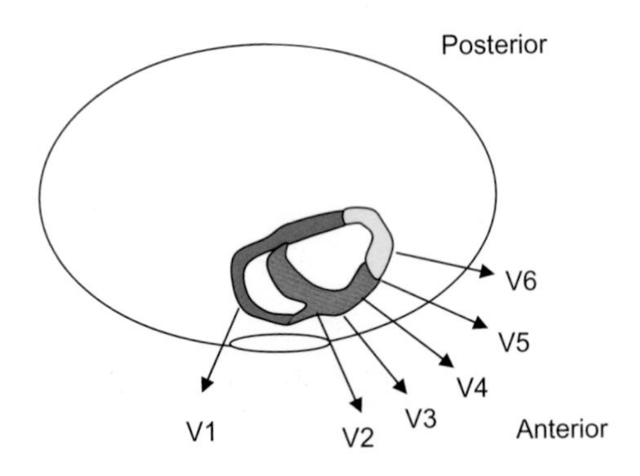

Figure 3.20 Localisation of chest leads

the echocardiography, you would expect regional wall motion abnormality/hypokinesia of the left lateral wall. On the angiogram, you would see critical stenosis of the affected vessel which in this case would be the circumflex artery.

Let's take another example, occlusion of the left anterior descending artery would lead to infarction of the area supplied by it: predominantly the anterior wall of the heart supplied by V2–4 (and often V5 and V6). Therefore, you would expect ST elevation on your ECG in those leads. A combination of involvement of both the anterior and lateral leads would suggest an anterolateral infarction. This may mean the there are stenoses of both the circumflex and LAD, or even involvement of the left main stem.

You will notice from the ECG (Fig. 3.21) that there is also ST depression in leads II, III and aVF. This phenomenon on the opposite wall from the wall which shows the prominent ST elevation, is known as **reciprocal changes**, and strongly supports the diagnosis of acute MI.

Table 3.5 summaries the corresponding 2D ECG changes with the location of the MI. Exactly which V leads are involved in which type of infarct is not critical to memorise, since arteries vary, but remember the concept that the low-numbered V leads map to the septum with V4 near the apex (all of which are generally LAD), and V5 and 6 continue past the apex and map to LAD or branches of the circumflex.

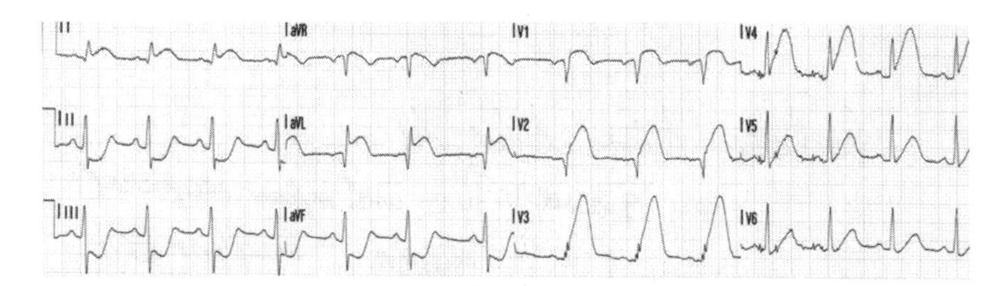

Figure 3.21 Anterolateral MI on ECG

Table 3.5 ECG changes and the location of infarction

Leads	ST change	Location	Arteries affected
V_{2-4}	Elevation	Septal or anterior	LAD
I, aVL	Elevation	Lateral	Circumflex
V_{2-6}, I, aVL	Elevation	Anterolateral	LAD with circumflex, or LMS on its own
II, III, aVF	Elevation	Inferior	Almost always supplied by RCA
V_{1-3}	Depression	Posterior	Circumflex or RCA (depending which supplies the posterior wall)

- **Full thickness (transmural) infarct.**
  - In the event of a significant MI where there is subsequent infarction and death of, for example, the anterior myocardial wall.
  - Dead myocardium produces no electrical output.
  - If there is no signal originating from the anterior myocardium, the only signal the anterior leads perceive is the normal signal from the myocardium at the opposite side of the heart, going away from the electrodes.
  - The net result is a **Q wave** — which is indicative as a late ECG change in this condition.

- **Posterior myocardial infarction.**
  - In this situation, the 'ST elevation' originates from posterior myocardium.
  - There are no electrode sensors on the back of the patient in a standard 12 lead ECG.
  - Therefore signals emitted from the posterior myocardium are recorded as going **away** from the anterior chest leads, giving upside down ST elevation — in other words, ST depression.
  - In patients with **deep ST depression anteriorly** with evidence of elevation elsewhere, consider posterior infarct.

3.4 ECG Examples

Please refer to the Appendix for examples of common ECG findings.

3.5 Exercise Tolerance Test (ETT)

ETT (Exercise ECG) is a 12-lead ECG recorded during a period of exercise with the patient on a treadmill. ETT often follows a 'Bruce protocol' which has progressively more demanding stages of 3 minutes each. Achieving 9 minutes of **Bruce protocol** is usually favourable. If a patient achieves less than 85% of their age-predicted target heart rate (220 bpm minus age in years), the test is considered to be non-diagnostic. There is a ***Modified Bruce*** protocol, which inserts an extra-gentle 'stage 0' before stage 1, to allow for very elderly, frail, or weak patients.

During exercise, the effect of the progressive increase in intensity (increased treadmill pace/slope) on conduction, heart rate and blood pressure is recorded.

3.5.1 *What are the indications for an exercise ECG?*

These include assessment of:

- Exercise tolerance
- Exercise-induced arrhythmias

- Response to treatment/prognostic indicators, that is, in angina/MI/cardiomyopathy

Mortality in ETT is 1 in 10,000. β-blocker and digoxin therapy are stopped at 1 and 7 days respectively as digoxin can cause a false positive test result.

3.5.2 *What is a 'Positive Test'?*

- Ischaemia-downward sloping ST depression >1 mm. Taking 0.5 mm increases the sensitivity and decreases the specificity.
- Excessive ST changes.
- Arrhythmia, that is, ventricular tachycardia (VT).
- Chest pain.

Commonest **reasons for stopping the test** are fatigue, SOB and a 'positive test' result.

Contra-indications: Acute MI (within 4–6 days), unstable angina (rest pain in the previous 48 hours), acute myo/pericarditis, aortic stenosis, and severe heart failure.

- ***Note*: The presence of left bundle branch block (LBBB) makes the results of the ETT difficult to interpret.**

3.6 Cardiac Imaging

The heart is an internal organ which lies within the mediastinum. Its location behind the ribcage and the scapula can limit its accessibility to direct imaging.

However, modern medicine has evolved to identify both invasion and non-invasive modalities for viewing and evaluating the function of the heart and its structures within the mediastinum.

The following pages cover some of these modalities including:

- Echocardiography (Echo)
- Myocardial perfusion imaging
- Multi gated acquisition scan — MUGA
- Coronary angiography
- Cardiac CT

3.7 Echocardiography (ECHO)

An echocardiogram is a non-invasive ultrasound assessment of the heart and vessels. It can provide useful information on the anatomy, haemodynamics and both the systolic and diastolic function of the heart.

It can be performed under resting conditions as a baseline assessment, or under controlled stress conditions to provide a functional assessment in valve or coronary artery disease. It can also help to rule out aortic dissection and pulmonary embolism.

3.7.1 *Echocardiography basics*

Echo utilises ultrasound technology and requires a transducer/probe to transmit the waves. It is usually made of a ***piezoelectric crystal*** — a crystal that deforms (ever so slightly) when a voltage is put across it. When you vary the voltage across it, you cause thickening and thinning of the transducer and a sound wave is created. The waves travel through the tissues and are reflected off tissue interfaces (for example, between blood and tissue). The reflected wave causes changes to the transducer which leads to changes in voltage that can be picked up as a signal and interpreted. The timing of the reflected waves gives an indication of depth of the underlying structure.

Ultrasound travels freely through fluid and soft tissues and are reflected back against more solid (dense) tissue. The resolution which is defined as the ability to differentiate small structures is roughly half of the wavelength of the sound wave which in turn is defined by the following relationship:

$$c = \lambda \times f$$

c is the velocity of the wave, λ is the wavelength and f is the frequency.

The standard wavelength frequency used in adult echocardiography is usually between 2.5–3MHz. This corresponds to a resolution of 0.3 mm (if c is approx 1540 m/s and wavelength therefore 0.6 mm). Resolution can be improved by increasing the frequency; however higher frequencies are less able to penetrate tissues.

Overlying bone and air yields poor images and patients with chronic obstructive lung disease with expanded lungs full of air are often difficult to scan. Gel placed between the probe and the patient improves the transmission of the waves.

3.7.2 *When should I request an Echo?*

- chest pain: to confirm a cardiac cause
- dyspnoea: to confirm/exclude a cardiac cause
- incidental murmur
- abnormal ECG
- cardiomegaly on CXR

3.7.3 *Types of scans*

- **M-mode *(motion mode)*:** single dimension (time) image produced on light sensitive paper moving at constant speed.
- **Two-dimensional *(real time)*:** 2D fan shaped image of the heart is produced. The four commonest views are subcostal, apical 4-chamber, parasternal long and short axis.
- **Doppler scan:** coloured jets illustrating flow and gradients across valves and septal defects.

A Doppler echocardiogram utilises the *Doppler principle* where the apparent frequency of the waves reflected off an object increases or decreases depending on whether the object is moving towards or away from the transmitter. In a patient, the frequency of blood that is flowing towards the transmitter will appear higher and likewise, the frequency of blood moving away from the transmitter will

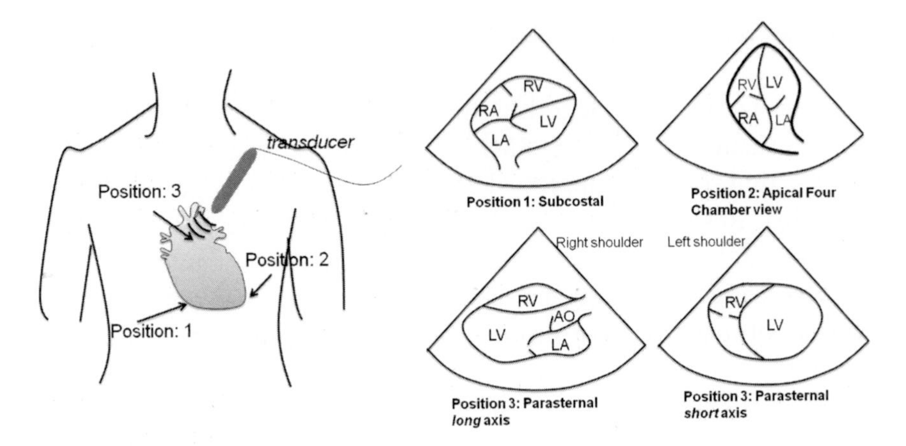

Figure 3.22 The four commonest views in transthoracic echocardiography. Adapted from http://faculty.ksu.edu.sa

appear lower. The difference between the original transmitted 'true' velocity and 'apparent' frequency can be used to calculate the velocity of blood flow. The blood flow is also represented by coloured jets indicating its direction either towards or away from the transmitter.

3.7.4 *What does this echocardiogram show?*

Below are five simple steps to interpreting an echocardiogram.

Step 1: Look at the ejection fraction (EF) and systolic function

An EF of <40% could indicate systolic heart failure, however it is important to remember that heart failure can occur in the presence of a normal ejection fraction (>50%) as EF doesn't consistently track the early stages of decline in ventricular function.

Step 2: Look for regional wall motion abnormalities

An old myocardial infarction is evidenced by regional wall motion abnormality and thinning.

Step 3: Looking for valvular heart disease

An echo is very useful in a patient who presents with a murmur as it can distinguish between those that are functional and those that indicate structural heart disease. If a valvular condition is identified, an echo can allow for quantification of the lesion, severity and assessment of function.

Step 4: Look at the measurement of LV wall thickness and mass

This is useful in a patient whose ECG shows left ventricular hypertrophy or right ventricular strain as well as an incidental finding of pathological Q waves to confirm the presence of an old transmural myocardial infarction (for more details see section on 'ECG').

Step 5: Look at the measurement of the heart size

Cardiomegaly can be due to a number of reasons including:

- left ventricular dilatation
- right ventricular dilatation
- atrial enlargement
- underlying valvular heart disease
- composite shadow from the lung without true cardiac abnormality

3.8 Stress Echocardiography

A stress echo is where is the heart is put under 'stress' conditions usually by injecting the patient with dobutamine just beforehand. As the conditions are made to emulate exercise, the patient may feel hot, sweaty and flushed. It may also cause angina, breathlessness and/or palpitations.

3.8.1 *Advantages over exercise ECG*

An echocardiogram is more useful than an exercise ECG in diagnosing ischaemia. This is because ECG abnormalities such as bundle branch block, left ventricular hypertrophy, non-specific ST segment or T wave abnormality can mask ischaemic changes on the ECG and make the test inconclusive. It can also stratify patients into different risk categories.

3.9 Transoesophageal Echocardiography (TOE)

Whereas transthoracic echocardiography (TTE) explained above has the advantage of being a non-invasive procedure, transoesophageal echo involves passing a transducer probe into the patient's oesophagus. As the oesophagus lies in direct contact with the heart, the advantage is that it can provide clearer images as well as Doppler evaluation of the heart.

3.9.1 *When should I request a TOE?*

- looking for source of emboli and vegetation in endocarditis
- assessing prosthetic valves
- diagnosing aortic dissection

TOE is a longer procedure, involves fasting and sedation of the patient.

TOE provides better clarity for structures near the back of the heart or back of the chest, including the aorta, coronary arteries, and the valves of the hearts.

3.9.2 *Side effects*

- oesophageal perforation (1 in 10,000)
- sedation causing aspiration or apnoea
- respiratory arrests or arrhythmias (a stocked resuscitation trolley should be available nearby)

3.9.3 *Contra-indications*

- oesophageal disease
- cervical spine instability

3.10 Myocardial Perfusion Scan (Thallium or MIBI Scan)

A myocardial perfusion scan is a nuclear scan looking at the blood flow within the heart. Like an exercise tolerance test, it has both a rest and stress element. A radioisotope, commonly thallium or technetium, is injected into a peripheral vein. It travels to the coronary arteries and images are taken with a special gamma camera of the heart at rest and after a period of exercise.

A myocardial perfusion scan looks at the blood flowing through the coronary arteries and is useful in the diagnosis of coronary artery disease. It can also be used to identify areas of reversibility (myocardium amenable to reperfusion as opposed to dead myocardium) following a myocardial infarction. This information can be used when planning coronary bypass grafting to target reperfusion to damaged regions within the myocardial wall that are reversible.

Note: 'MIBI' (2-Methoxy IsoButyl Isonitrile) scan, 'technetium scans' and 'thallium scans' are all examples of myocardial perfusion scans.

3.11 MUGA — Multi Gated Acquisition Scan

A MUGA scan is another radioisotope scan looking at how efficiently the heart is pumping. Again, a radioactive isotope, that is, technetium, is injected into a peripheral vein. The gamma camera is able to detect the technetium labeled cells and produces moving images of the heart. A MUGA scan can assess the degree of damage to the myocardium following a myocardial infarction. More importantly, it can give an accurate and reproducible assessment of left ventricular ejection fraction, a very useful indicator of cardiac function. It is used in patients undergoing chemotherapy to assess whether the drugs are having an adverse effect on cardiac function.

3.12 Coronary Angiography

Angiography is widely used in medicine in the diagnosis and management of a range of vascular conditions from head to toe.

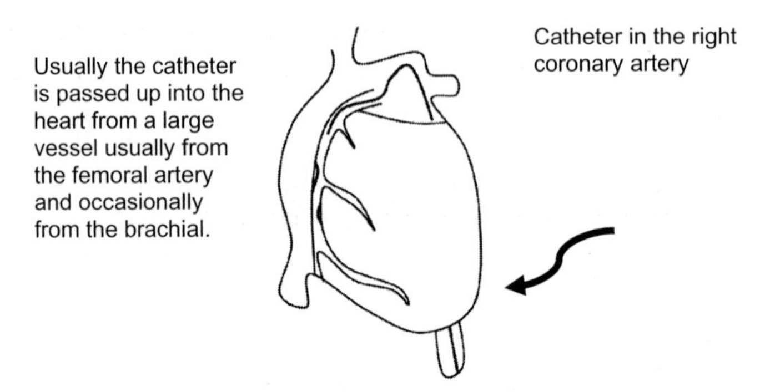

Figure 3.23 Catheter in a coronary artery

In cardiology, it has both diagnostic and therapeutic uses in coronary artery disease.

3.12.1 *How is an angiogram performed?*

The angiogram is performed in a catheterisation laboratory ('cath lab') and can be performed under local anaesthetic.

A catheter is introduced in either the femoral or radial artery and advanced around the aortic arch until it sits in the coronary artery. Through the catheter, a radio-isotope dye (contrast) is injected and real-time X-ray images can be taken of the moving blood in the coronary vessels. Narrowed sections within the arteries are thus visualised.

3.12.2 *What happens after the procedure?*

Back on the wards after the procedure, the arterial sheath is kept in for about 4 hours until the effects of the heparin has worn off. Patients are usually advised to lie flat for a couple of hours and ECG monitoring is maintained. Mild chest pain can occur during this time due to the stretching of the coronary adventitia and should resolve within a couple of hours. An increase or new onset chest pain can signify abrupt occlusion of the vessel which warrants immediate return to the cath lab for re-opening. In such a case, the ECG may pick up ST elevation or T wave changes. Patients can generally return to work after 5–7 days.

3.12.3 *What are the risks of the procedure?*

Risks:

General

- bleeding
- infection
- allergic reaction to the anaesthetic or contrast

Specific

- dislodgement of a clot inducing MI/stroke
- renal injury from contrast, usually transient
- death <1/1000

3.12.4 *What is an angioplasty?*

An *angioplasty* is the therapeutic dilatation of the narrowed coronary vessels. The first human angioplasty was performed in 1977 by Andreas Gruentzig. A balloon is introduced via the catheter which can be inflated to widen a stenosed section of the artery. It acts both to stretch the vessel wall as well as to longitudinally redistribute the atherosclerotic plaque. This is known as percutaneous transluminal coronary angioplasty (PTCA) and is associated with an average restenosis rate of 30–35%. Furthermore, the uncontrolled wrenching of the plaque can lead to an abrupt closure of the coronary artery in 5–8% of patients. Coronary stenting was introduced in the late 1980s and involves the placement of a 'scaffold' across the narrowed artery eliminating elastic recoil after angioplasty. Large randomised controlled trials (RCTs) have shown this measure to reduce the early ischaemic complications although 10–20% of patients still experience recurrent symptoms 12 months following stent implantation.

3.12.5 *When should a coronary angioplasty be performed?*

Coronary angioplasty can be done as an emergency procedure known as primary percutaneous coronary intervention (PCI) or an elective one in patients with longstanding coronary artery disease, congenital and/or valve disease.

While most angiography is done as an outpatient procedure, most elective angioplasties are currently done with an overnight stay after the procedure.

Which patients with coronary artery disease are suitable?

Patients with ST-elevation myocardial infarction (STEMI)

- Primary PCI is preferred over the use of fibrinolytics if the facilities are available as it provides a more rapid and complete reperfusion as well as a lower risk of mechanical complications (for example, ruptures).

Patients with no or mild angina

- Medical therapy preferable.

Patients with moderate or severe angina

- PCI recommended for these patients retaining a moderate to large area of viable myocardium.

Patients with unstable angina or Non-STEMI

- Evidence to show benefits with glycoprotein IIb/IIIa inhibitors and coronary stents.

3.12.6 *Special precautions*

Special precautions are required for the following patients:

- Patients on warfarin may need to stop these 2–3 days prior to the procedure due to risk of bleeding at the site of catheter insertion. Consider putting these patients on heparin.
- Diabetic patients will need clarification with the doctor as to when they should take their medication — follow the local hospital protocol.

3.12.7 *Primary percutaneous coronary intervention (PCI) versus thrombolysis*

Evidence from systematic reviews and meta-analyses show that primary percutaneous coronary intervention is superior to thrombolysis in the treatment of acute coronary syndromes with ST elevation. This benefit has been shown to be most effective within 12 hours of onset and independent of which thrombolytic agent used. It has been shown to reduce both short and long term mortality, stroke, reinfarction and need for coronary bypass graft surgery.

The use of drug eluting stents remains controversial. These are stents coated with immunosuppressive drugs such as sirolimus, everolimus and polymer-derived paclitaxel presumably to reduce the risk of restenosis. Long-term studies show, however, they may be associated with a greater risk of late stent thrombosis, requiring a more prolonged duration of clopidogrel to counteract this.

3.12.8 *Post-procedure*

Following an angioplasty patients need the appropriate antiplatelet therapy.

- For patients having undergone a primary PCI for acute MI, long-term aspirin 75 mg and clopidogrel 75 mg for one month is recommended.
- For patients having undergone a primary PCI for stable angina, long-term aspirin 75 mg is recommended.
- For patients who have drug eluting stents, long-term aspirin and clopidogrel are recommended for at least 12 months.

Under the regulations of the Driver and Vehicle Licensing Agency (DVLA), patients are advised not to drive for a week after an angioplasty for angina. After an MI, driving must cease for a month.

3.12.9 *What is the risk of restenosis post-procedure?*

Restenosis can occur in anywhere from 25–60% stents. The likelihood of restenosis depends not only on the target stenosis, but on concomitant risk factors such as diabetes.

3.12.10 *New developments in coronary angiography and angioplasty*

1. *Distal embolic protection devices* — This is to prevent distal embolisation following PCI. Some studies have shown that these devices reduce post-procedure complications in some settings; other studies have not confirmed this. There are three types, one involves distal occlusion using a balloon that trapped a stagnant column of blood and allows for aspiration of any debris before the stent is deployed. Another uses a filter to trap any liberated debris and the third type consists of a proximal occlusion of the vessel with a balloon whereby liberated debris can then be removed by the guiding catheter.
2. *Gene therapy* — There are currently some ongoing clinical trials on the use of gene therapy to grow new blood vessels or muscle cells in patients following a myocardial infarction, or even to prevent the clot forming in the first place.

3.13 CT Coronary Angiogram

For many years, the continuous motion of the heart made imaging with CT and MRI difficult. Advances in technology have made it possible to combine images from several cardiac cycles to produce a single high resolution image of the heart in both CT and MRI.

At the same time, the anatomical resolution obtainable by CT has improved significantly with the advent of the 64-slice CT machine. CT coronary angiography has the advantage over angiography of being a less invasive procedure with a lower risk of infection. Contrast is injected via a peripheral vein rather than a femoral catheter. The CT scan highlights the flow of the contrast through the vessels and defines any stenoses or blockage. The main disadvantage is, however, a greater exposure to

Table 3.6 Advantages and disadvantages of CT angiography

Advantages	Disadvantages
Quick	Radiation exposure greater than that for invasive angiography
Non-invasive	Expensive
Lower risk of infection	Operative dependent for interpretation
	Does not allow for therapeutic intervention
	Not as suitable for evaluating smaller vessels (due to lower spatial resolution)

radiation than with invasive angiography. It is also operator dependent and does not allow for therapeutic intervention.

There are 16-slice and 64-slice machines currently available with a 256-slice machine soon to follow. A single CT coronary angiogram is equivalent to about 3–6 years of background radiation, or 300–600 chest radiographs. As the anatomical resolution and availability of CT angiography increases, it's applications in clinical practice are likely to increase.

3.13.1 *Side effects*

- Severe allergic reaction with contrast occurs in 0.2–0.7% of patients

3.13.2 *Contra-indications*

- Patients with typical angina and strongly positive exercise ECG
- Patients with renal dysfunction
- Patients with known allergy to contract media
- Young patients with coronary risk factors

3.13.3 *Prior to procedure*

Blood tests and ECG should have been done. Patients are required to stop eating and drinking about 4 hours prior to the procedure. Patients for whom beta-blockers are not contra-indicated may be given metoprolol to decrease the heart rate which improves temporal resolution. Patients should also be encouraged to drink two glasses of water before the test.

3.13.4 *During the procedure*

With a 64-slice machine, patients are required to hold their breath for less than 10 seconds. This is to reduce motion artefact. Newer machines, such as the 256-slice machine, reduce the requirement. A non-ionic water soluble contrast is used and is usually injected into the right upper limb (providing the shortest pathway to the heart).

3.13.5 *Interpreting the data*

Radiologists or cardiologists can apply various post-processing tools to obtain the best imaging quality for a particular coronary artery or segment.

Assessment of graft patency

CT coronary angiography has found a niche in evaluating the patency of grafts of patients who have previously undergone CABG. Often such patients are elderly, and have co-morbidities. These features put them at high risk of complications from conventional coronary angiography, and therefore CT angiography allows some of them to avoid the procedure.

Calcium scoring

This is based on the assumption that calcium load is proportional to atherosclerotic build up in the coronary arteries. Calcium scoring can provide a strong prognostic value for the risk of future coronary events. The downfall is that the absence of calcium doesn't necessarily mean an absence of atherosclerosis.

Assessment of coronary stenosis

There are many methods to such an assessment including simple 'eyeball', direct measurement as well as making use of automated vessel analysis software programmes.

Stenosis should be assessed in two orthogonal views and judged by the size of their lumen rather than the size of the wall. A 50% stenosis is generally accepted as clinically significant although the coronary reserve flow is not affected until there is 70–75% stenosis.

In general, CT tends to overestimate the degree of stenosis. Other factors include operator variability and a difference in measurement and estimation techniques.

Chapter 4

Commonly Encountered Conditions

Attending outpatient clinics can be an extremely valuable learning experience. However, with increasing time restraints on senior staff, it is important to be proactive in making the most of the available opportunities. If you let it all float past, you can end up sitting in the corner while the clinic happens around you, catching the odd pathology 'here and there' without making the best of your opportunities to gain understanding and experience.

In this chapter we will explore the most commonly encountered conditions, thus enabling you to be better prepared to get the most out of your time in clinic. We recommend reading the chapters before the clinic sessions so that you can concentrate on improving the recognition of key symptoms and signs, examining the patient and understanding the current management protocol in both out and in-patient clinical settings.

Remember you are NOT expected to know everything there is to know about these conditions, but you will impress your seniors by demonstrating a practical knowledge of these common conditions.

4.1 Atherosclerosis

Atherosclerosis is a multifactorial, chronic inflammatory process characterised by the build-up of an *atheromatous plaque* which narrows the luminal diameter of an artery.

Let's begin by examining a 'normal' blood vessel — composed of endothelial cells. The endothelium has three layers: tunica intima, tunica media, and tunica adventia.

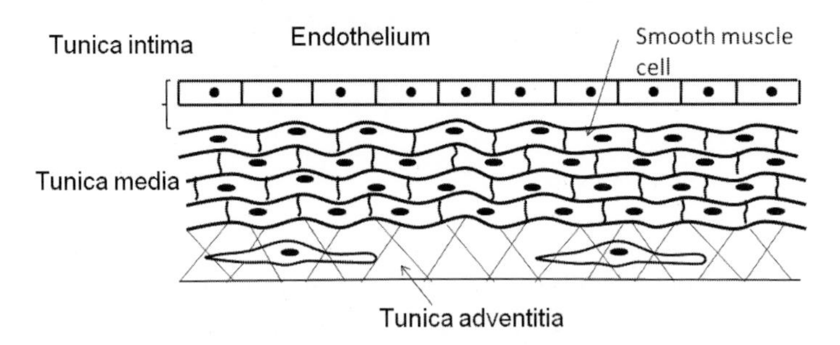

Figure 4.1 Layers of the endothelium

Five steps to understanding the pathogenesis of atherosclerosis:

1. **Damage to the arterial endothelium** — caused by repeated injury to the endothelial cells. This makes the endothelium more permeable to lipids and low density lipoprotein (LDL) allowing them to migrate into the tunica intima.
2. **Formation of a fatty streak** — macrophages are also 'attracted' to the injured endothelium and migrate into the intima. They then take up the oxidised LDL to form foam cells. The foam cells together with activated platelets trigger the movement of smooth muscle cells from the tunica media into the intima.
3. **Lipid plaque** — the build up of smooth muscle cells, foam cells and free lipids creates the lipid plaque.
4. **Fibrous plaque** — as the plaque grows, the smooth muscle cells are replaced by collagen. The collagen layer forms a fibrous plaque.
5. **Thrombus formation** — when the plaque fissures, this results in further platelet aggregation and the formation of a thrombus, causing further narrowing of the luminal diameter of the vessel.

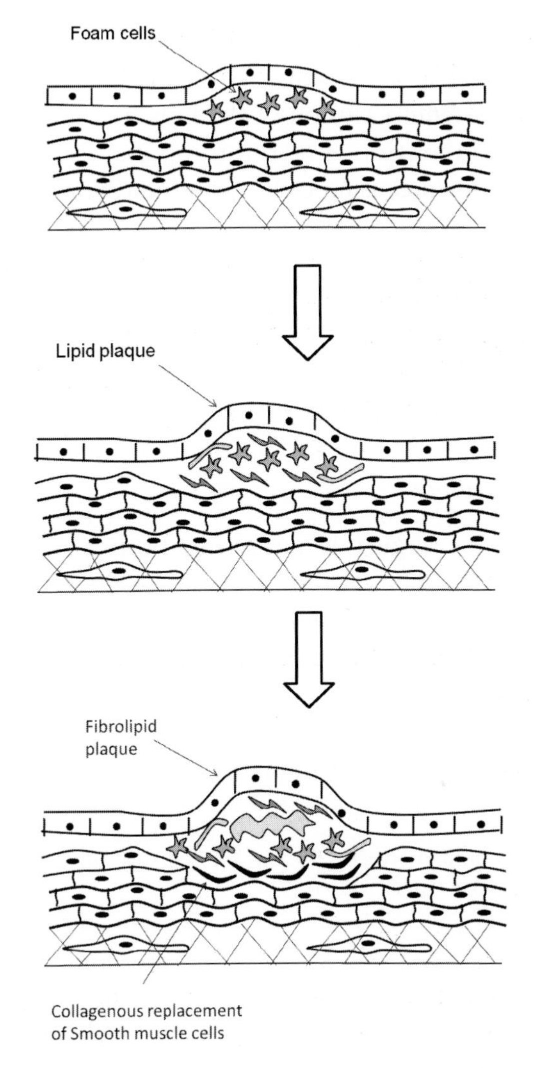

Figure 4.2 Formation of an atheromatous plaque

The plaque that forms has several clinical implications:

- **Stable angina** is caused by progressive stenosis (narrowing) of the vessel. This reduces the blood supply to the tissues during exercise/exertion known as *ischaemia* resulting in hypoxic damage to the cells causing pain.

- **Unstable angina** is due to acute fissuring and rupture of the plaque resulting in a thrombus that can cause *sub-total* occlusion of the lumen.
- **Myocardial infarction** is *total* thrombotic occlusion of the lumen causing cell death (infarction).

Part of the acute coronary syndromes

4.2 Angina

Angina pectoris is a Latin phrase meaning 'tight chest'. It is derived from the Greek word 'agkone' which means 'strangling'. The term 'angina' is used to describe chest pain due to *myocardial ischaemia.*

4.2.1 *Epidemiology*

The prevalence of angina is increasing both amongst males and females in the UK. The current estimate of affected individuals in the UK stands at approximately two million people! Contributory, non-modifiable factors include: increasing age and gender (angina is more common in males than females).

A prevalence snapshot is provided by the findings from the 2006 Health Survey for England (summarised below).

Percentage of patients between 55 and 64 years of age who have or have had angina:

- 8% of men
- 3% of women

Percentage of patients between 65 and 74 years of age who have or have had angina:

- 14% of men
- 8% of women

4.2.2 *Mechanism*

Myocardial ischaemia occurs when the myocardial blood supply is inadequate to meet the oxygen demand. Depicted below is a simple

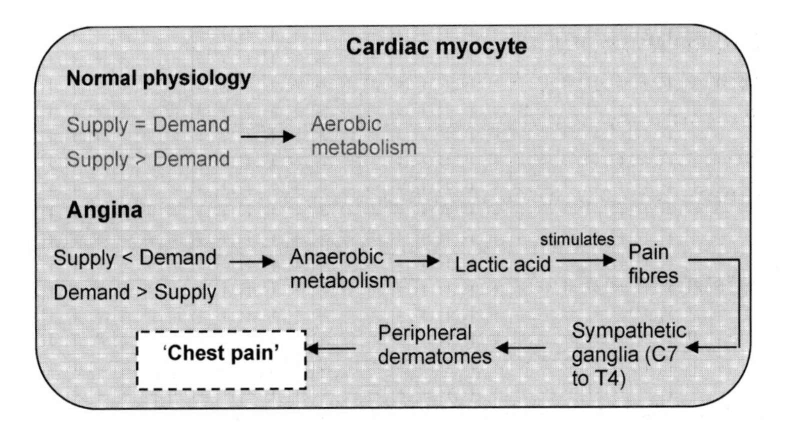

Figure 4.3 Complications of myocardial infarction

model illustrating both normal physiology, and the proposed mechanism of ischaemic chest pain at the cellular level.

4.2.3 *Causes of angina*

This can be classified using the '**supply**'/'**demand**' dichotomy.

1. Factors that **decrease supply** include:
   - *coronary atherosclerosis* — this is the commonest cause of angina and is due to narrowed vascular lumen, reducing the blood supply to the myocardium
   - coronary vasospasm
   - thrombus (blood clot)

2. Factors that **increase** the myocardial oxygen **demand** include:
   - **H**ypertension/hypertrophic cardiomyopathy (HCM)
   - **A**ortic stenosis/anaemia
   - **T**hyrotoxicosis/tachycardia
   - **E**xercise/exertion

Classification of angina

- **Stable angina** — 'predictable', chest pain on exertion, relieved by rest/glycerine trinitrate (GTN) spray/tablet.
- **Unstable angina** — 'unpredictable' angina with worsening frequency, and severity on minimal exertion/at rest. The risk of myocardial infarction (MI) if untreated is high (~ one in three patients will progress to have an acute MI). Unstable angina is also known as **crescendo angina**. Note: Unstable angina is part of the acute coronary syndromes (see ACS below).
- **Variant/Prinzmetal's angina** — due to coronary vasospasm. Chest pain occurs usually when the patient is at rest/asleep.
- **Decubitus angina** — angina at night whilst the patient is in the decubitus position, that is, lying down.

4.2.4 *History*

See Chapter 1 *Clerking patients.*

4.2.5 *Examination*

See Chapter 2 *Bedside teaching* for a step-by-step guide on examination.

4.2.6 *Investigations*

- **Blood tests** — full blood count (remember that anaemia is a cause of cardiac ischaemia/angina), urea and electrolytes, glucose, lipid profile, cardiac enzymes and troponin (see Chapter 3 *Investigations* for full details on when to take blood for troponin and how to interpret troponin levels). Liver function tests (LFT), and thyroid function tests (TFT) are also useful.
- **ECG** — look for evidence of left ventricular hypertrophy — also seen in hypertension and aortic stenosis (see the *Electrocardiography* section of Chapter 3 *Investigations*). Q waves may also be present — indicative of previous 'old' myocardial infarction. In contrast, unstable angina is often associated with dynamic ST segment changes (ST depression) +/– T wave inversion.
- **Chest radiograph** — usually normal, but may show cardiomegaly.

- **Exercise ECG** (Exercise Tolerance Test — see Chapter 3 *Investigations*)
  - o Most patients with angina/suspected angina will have this test.
  - o Sensitivity and specificity — depends on the patient cohort (higher in patients with triple vessel disease and lower in those with single vessel disease).
  - o A normal ETT does NOT exclude a diagnosis of angina.
  - o False positives are common in females.
- **Coronary angiography** — invasive but useful anatomy and severity indicator, particularly in high risk symptomatic patients. Also used to assess/evaluate valvular heart disease and left ventricular function.
- **Myocardial perfusion scan** — with a stressor, that is, exercise/adenosine or dobutamine. This is a non-invasive diagnostic investigation. Particularly useful:
  - o for females with low risk of cardiovascular disease but high risk of false positive ETT.
  - o prior to angioplasty to identify regional ischaemia.

Other investigations of use include: stress echocardiography, cardiac Magnetic Resonance Imaging (MRI), and cardiac computed tomography (CT). For more detail, please see Chapter 3 *Investigations.*

4.2.7 *Management of angina: acute 'stable' angina*

IMMEDIATE MANAGEMENT: '**symptom relief**' Sit patient up

↓

Stop precipitant, that is, exertion/eating

↓

Give glyceryl trinitrate (GTN) spray, that is, two puffs sublingual
(Relief is usually within 3 minutes.)

↓

Re-assess patient

Note: If attacks of angina are increasing in frequency/severity, and are not relived by GTN, consider alternative diagnosis (that is, an acute coronary syndrome — unstable angina/myocardial infarction — see below for management).

The immediate management aims to **relieve** the initial symptoms. It should be followed by measures that reduce the morbidity and mortality associated with myocardial ischaemia. You must address the secondary risk factors in order to reduce the risk of unstable angina and myocardial infarction (end-point of the atherosclerotic phenomena).

Address **secondary risk factors** with:

Lifestyle interventions
- smoking cessation advice
- exercise
- weight loss measures
- reduction in total fat and saturated fat intake

Pharmacological interventions
- aspirin
- lipid lowering agent — that is, statin
- blood pressure control (see the section later in this chapter on *Hypertension*)
- good glycaemic control

If there are no contra-indications, ensure that the patient is on **ABCD**.

A — **Aspirin** 75 mg od (↓risk of myocardial infarction)
B — **Beta-blocker** +/– (↓myocardial oxygen demand)
C — **Calcium channel blocker** (that is, Nifedipine/Diltiazem)
D — **vasoDilator** = Nitrates (that is, sublingual GTN — acute and prophylactically before exertion, Isosorbide mononitrate)

Others:

- **Nicorandil** — K+ channel activator, vasodilator
- **Ivabradine** — blocks the 'I_f' (funny) channel in the sino-atrial node. It can be used to lower the resting heart-rate in patients who are intolerant of beta-blockers.

4.3 Acute Coronary Syndromes (ACS)

Acute coronary syndrome is an umbrella term which encompasses a spectrum of clinical presentations of the same atherosclerotic disease process. It includes:

- ST-Elevation Myocardial Infarction (**STEMI**),
- Non-ST-Elevation Myocardial Infarction (**NSTEMI**) and,
- **unstable angina**.

Stable angina is not part of the acute coronary syndrome. Less than 1% of stable angina will transform into an acute myocardial infarction!

4.4 ST-Elevation Myocardial Infarction (STEMI)

This is caused by fissuring of the atherosclerotic plaque, thrombus formation and subsequently occlusion of the vessel. This leads to necrosis of the myocardium downstream to the blockage and manifests as ST elevation on an ECG.

4.4.1 *Rapid assessment of the patient*

The 'classical' presentation is with severe, central crushing chest pain which lasts more than 20 minutes associated with nausea, sweating and pallor. They can also present with arrhythmias, cardiac arrest or heart failure. Other forms of presentation including atypical chest pain are addressed in Chapter 1 *Clerking patients.*

4.4.2 *Investigations and management*

Management of a STEMI involves early diagnosis and prompt treatment following the ABC approach with primary attention to the **A**irway, **B**reathing and **C**irculation. Patients should be given 100% oxygen initially. Intravenous access should be established and bloods sent for full blood count (FBC), urea and electrolytes (U&Es), cardiac enzymes including troponin, lipid profile and glucose. An ECG monitor should be attached to the patient as soon as possible.

The aim of treatment in STEMI is to restore blood supply to the myocardium that has not sustained permanent damage. Drug therapy includes **300 mg aspirin orally**, pain relief in the form of an **opiate intravenously** and an **antiemetic**, such as, metoclopramide. Give two puffs of GTN sublingually and also consider a beta-blocker in the absence of contra-indications such as asthma or left ventricular failure.

The **ECG criteria** for an ST elevation MI are as follows:

- ST elevation **>1 mm** in two adjacent **limb leads**
- ST elevation **>2 mm** in two adjacent **chest leads**

In addition, the following also constitutes a STEMI:

- new onset left bundle branch block (LBBB)
- **posterior infarct with ST depression in V1–3**

The diagnosis of STEMI is made on the basis of history, ECG changes and elevation of biochemical markers.

Once a diagnosis is established, **the gold standard treatment** is **percutaneous coronary intervention (PCI)** where possible; otherwise **thrombolytics** such as streptokinase or tissue plasminogen activator can be used. The greatest benefit of PCI is seen within 12 hours of the onset of the symptoms, so **time is muscle**!

The ECG evolves with the progression of a myocardial infarction. **Q waves develop after 1 or 2 hours** and represent loss of viable myocardium. The **ST elevation will gradually diminish over time** and can take up to two weeks in an inferior MI. In the presence of a left ventricular aneurysm, it may remain elevated indefinitely. Over time, T wave inversion may also develop. The important thing to remember is that **an MI is dynamic**; therefore it is important to obtain serial ECGs to monitor the changes.

4.4.3 *Contra-indications to thrombolysis*

- previous haemorrhagic stroke
- stroke or cerebrovascular accident (CVA) within 6 months

- active internal bleeding
- aortic dissection
- recent major surgery or trauma
- bleeding disorder

4.4.4 *Post-reperfusion therapy*

Following percutaneous coronary intervention or thrombolysis, the patient will need anti-thrombotic therapy to keep the arteries open usually with low molecular weight heparin (LMWH) in addition to aspirin and clopidogrel. Consider also starting a beta-blocker and ACE inhibitor. Patients will need daily examination for complications, serial ECGs and cardiac markers over the next couple of days.

4.5 Non-ST-Elevation Myocardial Infarction (NSTEMI)

NSTEMI is caused by fissuring of the atherosclerotic plaque without complete occlusion of the artery, such as in a STEMI. The result is still an acute coronary syndrome where patients present with symptoms of an acute MI; however, instead of ST elevation on ECG, there may be **non-specific ST changes such as ST depression or T wave inversion**. In such a scenario, **a rise in troponin level** would lend to the diagnosis of a NSTEMI.

4.5.1 *Management of NSTEMI*

The initial treatment of NSTEMI is the same as that of a STEMI. Always start with attention to **A**irway, **B**reathing and **C**irculation. Give the patient 100% oxygen initially. Ensure venous access and send blood for full blood count (FBC), urea and electrolytes (U&Es), cardiac enzymes including troponin, lipid profile and glucose. Again, an ECG monitor should be attached as soon as possible.

The diagnosis is dependent upon the clinical history, serial ECG changes and a rise in cardiac enzymes. The aim of treatment in this case is to prevent new thrombus formation which may exacerbate the extent of myocardial damage and reduce myocardial oxygen demand.

Give **aspirin 300 mg orally, clopidogrel 300 mg, a beta-blocker and low molecular weight heparin (LMWH).** At a later stage, Percutaneous Coronary Intervention (PCI) may also be considered.

4.6 Unstable Angina (UA)

This is a difficult diagnosis to make as the ECG may be normal **and** there is no elevation of cardiac enzymes.

However, the characteristics of unstable angina are:

- angina on effort of increasing frequency provoked by progressively less and less exertion
- angina occurring unpredictably without exertion
- a prolonged, unprovoked episode of chest pain

Patients with unstable angina are at high risk of further thrombotic event and therefore need to be treated as per the NSTEMI pathway above.

All patients with STEMI should subsequently be managed on a coronary care unit (CCU). Patients with NSTEMI/UA should be stratified into high or low risk groups depending on the history, clinical findings, ECG and cardiac enzyme changes. All patients need serial ECGs and cardiac enzymes and continuous ECG monitoring.

4.6.1 *Complications of acute coronary syndromes*

It is important to consider the likely causes in relation to the time since the presentation of symptoms. Therefore, complications should be categorised into those occurring **hours**, **days** or **weeks** following an acute myocardial infarction.

Table 4.1 Complication of myocardial infarction

Hours	Hours/Days	Days/Weeks
• Ventricular arrhythmias	• Cardiac rupture	• Thromboembolis
• Failed reperfusion	• Reinfarction	• Chronic heart failure
	• Ventricular septal tachycardia	• Ventricular defect
	• Papillary muscle rupture — mitral regurgitation	• Dressler's syndrome
	• Left ventricular rupture	

Dressler's syndrome: an autoimmune pericarditis that has a usual onset of 4–6 weeks post-MI.

However, when stumped for an answer on the complications of an acute MI, refer to the following mnemonic:

Spread

S — sudden death, shock — hypovolaemia/cardiogenic shock
P — pericarditis
R — rupture of papillary muscle/left ventricular free wall. May result in ventricular septal defect/mitral regurgitation
E — embolism (thromboembolism/thrombus)
A — arrhythmias and left ventricular aneursym
D — Dressler's syndrome

4.6.2 *Long-term management of acute coronary syndromes*

Patients should be encouraged to stop smoking, undertake regular exercise, and eat a healthy diet. In addition, *all* **patients should be on aspirin, beta-blocker, ACE inhibitor, and statin in the long term unless contra-indicated**.

4.7 Atrial Fibrillation (AF)

Atrial fibrillation (AF) is the most commonly sustained arrhythmia. So you are very likely to come into contact with a patient suffering from this on the ward or in clinic.

4.7.1 *The ABC approach to a patient with AF*

Whether you are in an exam, or suddenly called to see a patient on the ward, remember that there are three key factors necessary for the effective management of patients in AF.

They are:

- **A** — AF? — Confirm the diagnosis of AF by feeling the pulse. Remember patients with the paroxysmal form may not be in AF at the time of examination. Review the ECG (if it is irregularly irregular with no visible P waves then this is AF).
- **B** — Because? Why is this patient in AF? Are there any predisposing factors, that is, hypertension or infection? Consider the possible causes of AF (see below). Is it new onset (<48 hours) or old (>48 hours)?
- **C** — Look for, and address, the complications of AF (mainly thromboembolism, that is, stroke/transient ischaemic attack [TIA] or heart failure).

This simple approach will guide your history, examination, investigation and management.

Atrial fibrillation — FACTS:

Prevalence of AF (three key facts):

1. increases with age
2. approximately 1% in those over 60 and 10% in those over 80
3. it tends to be more common in men than women

AF is a major risk factor for *thromboembolic stroke*: 15% of patients with stroke are found to have concomitant AF. The principal site of thrombus formation is in the left atrial appendage. This is best visualised with a trans-oesophageal echocardiography (TOE).

- **ECG** — the hallmarks of atrial fibrillation on ECG are:

1. Irregularly irregular — QRS complexes occur at irregular times
2. No P waves (wavy baseline doesn't count)

- **Chest radiograph** — look for infection, pulmonary oedema or retrosternal goitre.
- **Urinalysis** — look for features of infection, such as, nitrites +/– leukocytes.
- **Echocardiography** — to assess cardiac function/structure.

4.7.7 *Management of atrial fibrillation*

Firstly, let's briefly explore some of the proposed mechanisms underpinning the development of the fibrillating atrium.

Pathogenesis of atrial fibrillation:

1. **Ectopic foci** — foci of atrial tissue commonly found at the site of the *pulmonary veins* can generate multiple ectopics leading to fibrillation (this is the reasoning behind pulmonary vein isolation — below).
2. **Multiple re-entry circuits** — arrhythmia in the chronic state is sustained by multiple re-entry and dividing wavelets colliding into each other.
3. **Tissue remodelling** — various conditions can cause the structure of the atrial tissue to be changed so that it is less favourable to sustaining normal sinus rhythm, and is instead more favourable to sustaining the multiple re-entrant circuits of atrial fibrillation. These conditions include hypertension, valve disease (especially mitral), myocardial infarction, and heart failure of any cause. The exact mechanism is unclear, but may involve a combination of left atrial dilatation (and stretch of individual myocytes), development of fibrous tissue replacing some atrial myocardium, and changes in the electrical properties of the atrial cells.

Three important distinctions:

Paroxysmal AF	Persistent AF	Permanent AF
Recurrent AF lasting minutes to hours, (<7 days) generally self-terminates within 48 hours.	AF that lasts for greater than 7 days requiring electrical or pharmacological cardioversion.	When attempts to restore sinus rhythm have been abandoned.

Principles of management:

1. **Rate** control.
2. **Rhythm** control — restoration of sinus rhythm by cardioversion either pharmacologically or electrically.
3. **Prevention of thromboembolic** events with anticoagulation.
4. Radiofrequency ablation — for refractory cases.

4.7.8 *Cardioversion*

The decision whether or not to cardiovert a patient is significantly influenced by the **haemodynamic status of the patient**, and the **onset of AF**. Is the patient haemodynamically stable? AF >48 hours onset?

No

Electrical (direct current) cardioversion (65–90% successful)

Main considerations are:

- need for sedation
- anticoagulation
- must have temporary pacing facilities at hand

Yes

Pharmacological cardioversion (successful if initiated within 2–7 days of onset)

- Flecainide
- Propafenone
- Amiodarone

4.7.9 *Pharmacological cardioversion — which drugs?*

Propafenone and **Flecainide** have a cardioversion rate of 75–80% within 3 hours.

Relapse following initial cardioversion = 25–50% in one month!

Note: Do **not** use in patients with known previous myocardial infarction/ischaemia, significant left ventricular systolic dysfunction, or bundle branch block (especially if 'trifascicular'). Flecainide may cause complete heart block necessitating temporary pacing!

Second line agent is **Amiodarone** with a cardioversion rate of 60–70%. It is, however, *safe* for use in patients with a *previous history of cardiac disease* hence it can be first line if any of the above contra-indications exist.

4.7.10 *Rhythm control*

Maintenance of rhythm control can be achieved with the following anti-arrhythmics (Vaughn-William classification — see Chapter 5 *Drugs*):

- class Ia (quinidine and disopyramide),
- class Ic (**flecainide** and **propafenone**), or
- class III (**sotalol** and **amiodarone**)

Remember all anti-arrhythmics are pro-arrhythmics!

There is an **increased risk** of fatal polymorphic ventricular tachycardia (*torsades de pointes*) with the use of class 1a, Ic drugs and sotalol. So don't forget to perform a 12 lead ECG at ~7 days, looking for the following ECG changes: prolonged QRS complex or QT interval.

4.7.11 *Rate control*

Commonly used agents work by increasing atrioventricular (AV) nodal blockade of the AF impulses:

- **Digoxin** — especially useful in sedentary patients (elderly).

- **Beta-blockers** (atenolol, bisoprolol, propranolol, metoprolol, and sometimes esmolol — very short acting).
- **Calcium channel blockers** (verapamil and diltiazem — the non-dihydropyridine calcium blockers) preferred in patients with obstructive airway disease, e.g., bronchial asthma, who may not tolerate beta-blockers.

Note: **Digoxin does not provide adequate control of heart rate during exercise**, and therefore it is usually reserved for elderly patients with sedentary lifestyles. In younger patients, combination therapy may be necessary.

To Impress!

Recent evidence from randomised trials (AFFIRM, PIAF, RACE and STAF trials — see abbreviations) have shown that **rate control is as effective as rhythm control** in improving symptoms and functional capacity in patients, particularly those over 65 years of age.

The AFFIRM trial recruited the largest number of patients (n = 4,060), who were randomised either to rate control with Digoxin, standard Beta blockers, Diltiazem and Verapamil, or to a strategy of obtaining and maintaining sinus rhythm using Amiodarone, Sotalol, Propafenone, and Flecainide. The mean follow up period was 3.5 years. Mortality rates were not significantly different between the two groups, but there was a trend towards more strokes in the rhythm control group due to discontinuation of anticoagulation on regaining sinus rhythm.

4.7.12 *Anticoagulation*

Patients with the following risk factors are considered high risk patients and should be on anticoagulant therapy unless contra-indicated.

Risk factors for thromboembolism in atrial fibrillation:

- Older age (although this is of course a continuous variable, thresholds of 60, 65 and 75 are sometimes used in scoring systems)

- Hypertension
- Diabetes mellitus
- Previous stroke/*TIA
- Structural heart disease
- Left ventricular dysfunction, vascular or ischaemic heart disease
- Hyperthyroidism
- Prosthetic valve.

Overall fivefold increase risk of stroke in patients with AF!
Note: **Loss of atrial systole decreases cardiac output by 20% which predisposes to thrombus formations.**

Table 4.2 Anticoagulation in AF: CHADS2 score

		Score
CHADS2 score		
C	Congestive cardiac failure	1 point
H	Hypertension	1 point
A	Age >75 years	1 point
D	Diabetes	1 point
S	Previous stroke/TIA*	2 points

Total score **≥3 (high risk)** ~6% risk of stroke per year (warfarin is indicated).
Total score <3 (moderate-low risk) 4% risk of stroke per year (consider warfarin or aspirin).

*TIA — transient ischaemic attack — focal neurological event resolving within 24 hours.

In a young patient with no risk factors or when warfarin cannot be given, aspirin is a reasonable alternative.

4.7.13 *Radiotherapy/Cryoablation therapy*

Radiofrequency and cryoablation therapy is generally reserved for the younger patient with a **structurally normal heart** with atrial fibrillation. These procedures are done by electrophysiologists and involve the use of radiofrequency ablation to isolate the pulmonary veins or other sites of ectopic focus (see *Pathogenesis of atrial fibrillation* — above). The procedure carries the risk of pulmonary vein stenosis and more importantly — systemic embolism. So a transoesophageal echo (TOE) is performed at the start to look for thrombus in the left atrial appendage. On completion, patients are discharged home on warfarin.

4.7.14 *The surgical alternative*

The **surgical maze** procedure employs the use of conduction blocks created either by incision or ablation in the atria to divert the flow of abnormal conduction. The risks involved are similar to the risks associated with **open heart surgery**.

4.7.15 *Discussion points and new developments*

There is recent evidence to indicate that statins, ACE inhibitors and angiotensin receptor antagonists may have a role in preventing recurrence in new onset atrial fibrillation (for example, LIFE trials).

New anticoagulants

New anticoagulants are currently being researched such as dabigatran and rivaroxaban thrombin inhibitors. In addition, the effectiveness of aspirin and clopidogrel in anticoagulation is being compared to the use of warfarin and aspirin alone.

New anti-arrhythmics

Areas of research and anticipated modes of action for proposed new anti-arrhythmics include:

- Stretch receptor antagonists
- Gap junction modulators
- Multi-channel blockers

- Adenosine analogues
- Agents with highly selective action on ion channels.

Surgery

More than 90% of thrombi form in the left atrial appendage. A new technique called Percutaneous Left Atrial Appendage Transcatheter Occlusion (PLAATO) involves inserting a self-expanding device in the left atrial appendage under fluoroscopic and transoesophageal echocardiographic guidance. Long-term efficacy and safety of this device is currently being investigated.

4.8 Other Arrhythmias

Arrhythmias or 'abnormal heart rhythms' are common. As there are many different types, it is important that you understand the principles of management. Here is a simple but practical way to classify arrhythmias based on:

- **Rate** — tachyarrhythmia (pulse >100 bpm) or a bradyarrhythmia (pulse < 60 bpm)?
- **QRS complex** — broad (> 120 ms) or narrow (<120 ms)? For example, a narrow complex tachyarrhythmia could be sinus tachycardia, atrial tachycardia, atrial flutter or fibrillation.

Rate and QRS complexes are the simplest and most useful way of classifying arrhythmias however Table 4.3 (below) contains other useful terminologies/classification that you may come across.

Let's begin by defining a common term used to classify arrhythmias: supraventricular tachycardia (SVT).

4.8.1 *Supraventricular tachycardia (SVT)*

The term 'supraventricular tachycardia' refers to a tachycardia arising above the ventricles. It is a narrow complex rhythm and can be subdivided into two further categories depending on where the action potential originates.

- Atrial tachycardias arise in the atrium and includes:
  - atrial fibrillation (AF) and,
  - atrial flutter.
- Junctional tachycardias arise at the atrioventricular node (AVN) and includes:
  - atrioventricular nodal re-entry tachycardias (AVNRT) and,
  - atrioventricular re-entry tachycardias (AVRT).

Table 4.3 Classification of arrhythmias

Types of arrhythmias		Examples
Supra ventricular tachycardia (SVT)	**Ectopic beats**	**Atrial ectopics** — random complexes with abnormal P waves
	Atrial arrhythmias	**Atrial fibrillation** — see above **Atrial flutter** — 'saw tooth' baseline, flutter wave **Atrial tachycardia** — fast with discrete abnormal P waves **Sinus tachycardia** — 'normal' but fast ECG
	Junctional arrhythmias	**Atrio-ventricular re-entry tachycardia (AVRT)** **Atrio-ventricular node re-entry tachycardia (AVNRT)**, that is, Wolff-Parkinson-White (WPW) syndrome
Ventricular arrhythmias		**Ventricular ectopics** — abnormal QRS complex **Ventricular tachycardia** — pulse >100 bpm with broad 'regular' QRS complexes **Ventricular fibrillation** — **medical emergency!** HR >100 bpm with irregular QRS complexes
Heart block (see chapter on *Investigations — ECG*)		**First degree** — prolonged PR interval **Second degree:** • **Mobitz type I (Wenckebach)** — prolonging PR interval with non-conducted P waves • **Mobitz type II** — normal PR interval with non-conducted P waves **Third degree** — complete dissociation of atrial and ventricular activity

4.8.2 *Speed of conduction through the myocardium*

Let's think about the speed of conduction, in general it can be:

- **Slow** — this occurs when the atrio-ventricular node acts as a pacemaker, that is, in **nodal** arrhythmias.
- **Medium** — when the **atrial or ventricular myocardium** acts as a pacemaker.
- **Very fast** — when the **His-Purkinje myocardium** acts as a pacemaker.

4.8.3 *How do I approach this patient?*

Again as in 'atrial fibrillation', the '**ABC**' approach is used here.

- **A** — Arrhythmia? — Is this patient really having an arrhythmia? Try to confirm your suspicions clinically. Take a focused history, examine the patient, and **do not forget to feel for the pulse**! Review the ECG/cardiac monitor (see chapter on 'Investigations' for details on how to read and interpret ECGs).
- **B** — Because? **Why** is this patient's heart beat abnormal? Are there any predisposing factors, that is, ischaemic heart disease, electrolyte abnormalities, drugs? Consider the possible causes (see below).
- **C** — Look for, and address, the complications of the arrhythmia. Is the patient compromised (**well or unwell?**) with the arrhythmia? Features of compromise include — chest pain, pulmonary oedema and shock/collapse.

4.8.4 *Causes of arrhythmias*

Here are the three commonest causes (if you re-arrange the first letters '**DIE**' is spelt).

- **I**schaemic heart disease
- **E**lectrolyte abnormalities
- **D**rugs.

Table 4.4 Others causes of arrhythmias

Cardiac	Non-cardiac	
• Cardiac insult, that is, post-myocardial infarction, cardiac surgery	• Drugs — anti-arrhythmics, caffeine, cocaine • Infection and pulmonary embolism (PE)	Common
• Inflammation — pericarditis/myocarditis • Cardiomyopathy • Cardiac surgery	• Thyroid disease • Exercise • Sick sinus syndrome • Genetic — that is, Brugada syndrome (see appendix) • Congenital, that is, Romano ward and Lange Nielsen Jevell syndrome (see *Appendix*)	↓
		Rare

4.8.5 *History*

The patient may be asymptomatic or present with any of the following symptoms:

- Palpitations or 'pounding in the chest'
- Syncope or presyncopal episodes — 'dizziness, fainting'
- Breathlessness
- Chest discomfort or pain
- Fatigue
- Stokes-Adams attacks (transient syncope caused by loss of cardiac output).

It is important that you understand and define **what, when, how and where** these symptoms occur. What impact do they have on the patient? Are there any precipitants or triggers? Have they ever resulted in loss of consciousness? At this point, it is worth re-visiting the first chapter for detailed exploration of these symptoms. **Ask the patient if they have been diagnosed with an arrhythmia before or have any ECGs with them?** For example, some patients with Wolff-Parkinson-White syndrome carry copies of their ECGs with them.

4.8.6 *Examination*

See Chapter 2 *Bedside teaching* for full details. Always start with a general inspection (from the end of the bed):

- **Does the patient look unwell?**
- Is this patient **HAEMODYNAMICALLY COMPROMISED?**
  - Look for features of hypoperfusion:
    - hypotension, that is, systolic BP < 90 mm Hg
    - low urine output
  - Pulmonary oedema
  - Cardiac ischaemia, e.g., chest pain
  - Reduced conscious level

If the answer to the above questions is 'Yes' then you are in an emergency and urgent steps are required (see management).

If 'No' then continue by looking for **signs** that may indicate the underlying cause, that is, heart disease, infection, or thyroid dysfunction (see 'atrial fibrillation'). Does the patient have any obvious neurological deficits suggesting a stroke or features of venous thromboembolism?

4.8.7 *Investigations*

As for 'atrial fibrillation' (see above), and includes:

- 12-lead ECG
- blood — including electrolytes, infectious screen, drug levels
- 24-hour holter monitor or 'tape'.

+/− event recorder, that is, a 'Reveal device', exercise ECG, echocardiography, cardiac catheterisation, electro-physiology study (EPS), and Tilt test.

4.8.8 *Management of arrhythmias*

General principles

Call for help! Whilst waiting for help to arrive, begin with the following five steps:

The 5-step immediate management plan

Step 1: Assess **haemodynamic status** — blood pressure, signs of heart failure, urine output, and level of consciousness.
Step 2: Print the **ECG** — you must try to capture the rhythm.
Step 3: Large bore **intravenous access** (very important!).
Step 4: Look for **cause**:

- Send blood including electrolytes — potassium, magnesium and calcium levels.
- Review the drug chart for causative agents.

Step 5: Ensure that the **crash trolley** is nearby!

4.8.9 *Using anti-arrhythmics drugs*

Adenosine — narrow complex tachycardia, diagnosis uncertain. Consider adenosine bolus (e.g., 6 mg whilst printing an ECG!) to see if it terminates or affects the rate. This may reveal an SVT or flutter with '**aberrancy**' (broad complex tachycardia-BCT) in sinus rhythm, that is, BCT with bundle branch block). As it is short acting it can be used in a 'diagnostic' fashion with BCTs.

Do not treat 'aberrant' rhythms with verapamil unless you are **certain** it is a supra-ventricular tachycardia (SVT) — it is **not safe** and may precipitate life threatening arrhythmia (see Wolff-Parkinson-White syndrome).

Management in special patient groups:

Patients with an ICD (implantable cardiac defibrillator) or pacemaker: discuss with a senior about contacting the pacing technician/cardiac physiologist with a view to trying overdrive pacing or Anti-Tachycardia Pacing ('command' ATP).

4.8.10 *Management of bradyarrhythmias*

Bradyarrhythmias include: sinus bradycardia, sinus node disease/sick sinus node (failure of the sinus node), heart block and junctional bradycardia (AV node acts as pacemaker when sinus node fails).

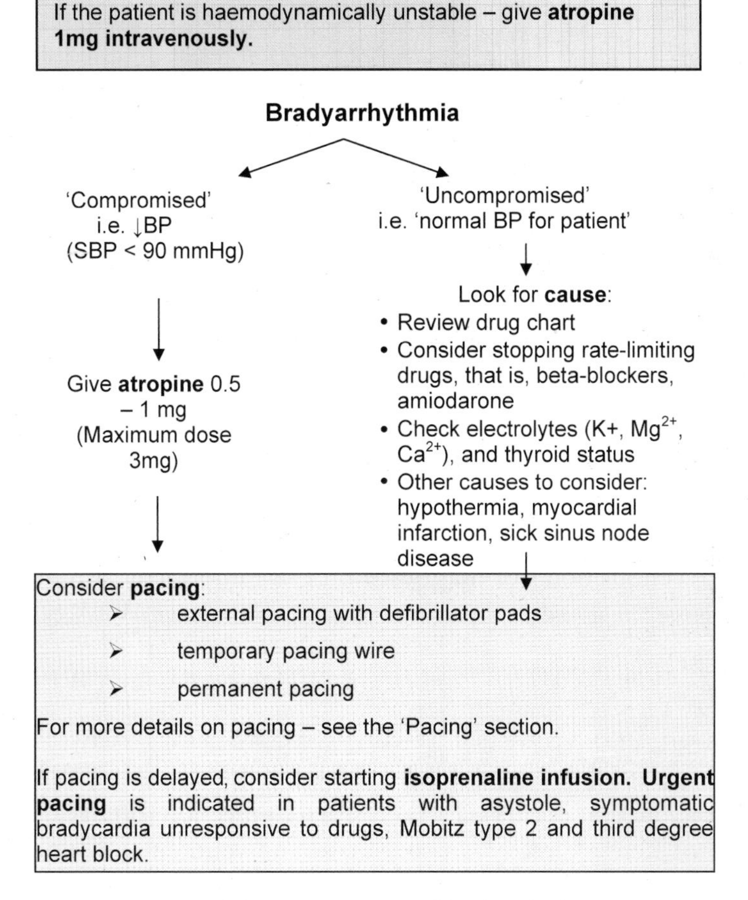

Figure 4.4 Management of bradyarrhythmia

4.8.11 *Management of tachyarrhythmias*

If the patient is haemodynamically unstable then cardiovert (**D**irect **C**urrent cardioversion) under sedation or general anaesthesia.

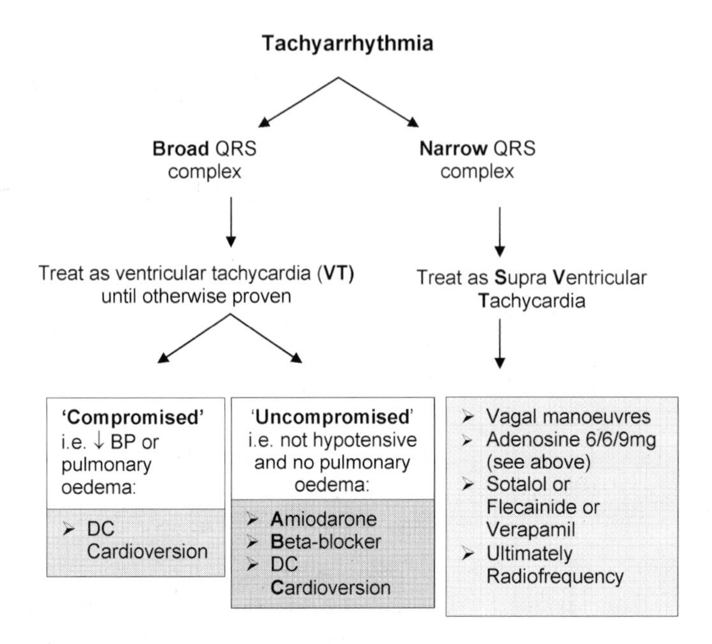

Figure 4.5 Management of tachyarrhythmia

- **Lignocaine** — may be used to treat ventricular tachycardia (in the absence of severe LV dysfunction) — discuss with senior. It is relatively short acting.
- Intravenous bolus of **magnesium** (4–8 mmol) may also help.
- If possible, avoid iv digoxin and verapamil — see WPW below.

4.8.12 *What is Wolff-Parkinson-White syndrome (WPW)?*

This is an atrio ventricular re-entry (reciprocating) tachycardia — AVRT — that is, it requires conduction via an accessory pathway. In WPW conduction occurs via an accessory connection (often called 'the bundle of Kent') directly between atrial and ventricular myocardium, situated somewhere around the AV rings.

4.8.13 *How is WPW diagnosed?*

On ECG, look for:

- **Short PR interval —**
  Conduction from the atrium to the ventricle (antegrade conduction) produces a short PR as the (slower) AV node is 'bypassed'

thus activating the ventricle earlier than expected, followed by 'medium' speed (slower than His-Purkinje and thus *broad QRS*) myocardial conduction.

- **Delta wave (slurring)**
  This is formed as the broad QRS merges with the narrow complex from the His/Purkinje-activated wavefront.

4.8.14 *How is WPW managed?*

Find out if the patient is aware that he or she has WPW or has been given an ECG of their arrhythmia (helpful especially if no previous ECG is available). Prior knowledge is useful as drugs that target the accessory pathway like flecainide may be effective if AV nodal blockers fail (see management of tachyarrhythmias — above).

Treatment of AVRT is the same as for any SVT (see above) with *some notable exceptions.* Avoid the use of adenosine or verapamil as it may lead to atrial fibrillation which can conduct rapidly over the accessory pathway resulting in a very fast ventricular rate and subsequent ventricular fibrillation. **Amiodarone, procainamide and cardioversion** are 'safer' alternatives. Definitive treatment is via **radiofrequency ablation** of the accessory pathway (see Atrial Fibrillation).

4.9 Hypertension

Lowering blood pressure by any means is one of the simplest means to prevent or retard the development of vascular disease. So critical is it that in many countries (including the UK) general practitioners have strict targets to detect and treat any elevation above national standards. If we ignore blood pressure when patients come to hospital we are undermining the interventions that are most likely to save most patients' lives.

It is increasingly clear that people with higher blood pressure have higher risk of heart attack and stroke, with no genuine threshold level of blood pressure at which risk rises particularly sharply: it just rises faster and faster as blood pressure rises further (an exponential rise).

Previous generations of doctors considered hypertension a disease, and therefore required a threshold level for diagnosis. Modern awareness of biology and current clinical practice recognises that there is no threshold, but that for practical purposes, thresholds help in selecting patients in whom we should make the effort to lower blood pressure.

The threshold for the definition of hypertension, in accordance with the British Hypertension society, European guidelines and World Health Organisation is a SBP ≥ 140–159, and a DBP ≥ 90–99.

4.9.1 *Blood pressure — understanding the basics*

It is the pressure difference (with high pressure at the left ventricle) that enables blood to flow from the aorta to the rest of the body and to return via the vena cava to the right atrium (low pressure).

Flow = pressure difference/resistance (where vessel resistance is dependent on the viscosity of the fluid and vessel dimension). Consequently small changes in vessel diameter will result in large increases in resistance, so the smaller the vessel diameter, the

Table 4.5 Factor affecting blood pressure

Factors affecting	
Peripheral Vascular Resistance	• Vasoconstrictors ○ Angiotensin and catecholamines (α and β adrenoceptors, that is, adrenalin) ○ Neural factors including hypoxia and pH • Vasodilators — prostaglandins
Cardiac Output	• Salt — sodium (Na+) • Hormones — aldosterone, anti-diuretic hormone (ADH) • Cardiac — heart rate, contractility

greater the resistance to flow. This is why vascular smooth muscle within the walls of the blood vessel has an important role to play in regulating the vessel diameter and hence the resistance to flow (blood pressure).

Thus an increase in Peripheral Vascular Resistance (PVR) +/− an increase in Cardiac Output (CO) will result in a higher blood pressure.

$$\uparrow \text{PVR} \quad \text{and/or} \quad \uparrow \text{CO} \quad \rightarrow \quad \uparrow \mathbf{BP}$$

Adjusting these factors allows us to exert some control over the blood pressure — see *Management* (below) for full details.

4.9.2 *What causes hypertension?*

In over 90% of patients, no single specific cause is found. This is known as 'Primary' hypertension. The presumed cause is usually multifactorial and involves a complex interplay of genetic and environmental factors. For example — epidemiological studies have confirmed ethnic variations in blood pressure, with many showing higher readings in blacks compared to whites.

However, in a small minority of patients (~5%), elevated BP readings may be '**secondary**' to a specific cause. The conscientious student/Doctor searches for and tries to exclude these by conducting a focused history, examination and investigation.

For causes of secondary hypertension — think **RED**:

Renal disease

Renal causes of elevated BP can be simplified using age:

Elderly	• Chronic renal failure
	• Renal artery stenosis
Very young	• Tumour, e.g., Wilm's nephroblastoma
All others	• Glomerulonephritis
	• Adult Polycystic Kidney Disease (autosomal dominant, so ask about family history of renal/pancreatic/liver cysts and subarachnoid haemorrhage)

- Chronic pyelonephritis
- Renal artery stenosis.

Remember that renal artery stenosis is secondary to atherosclerosis in the elderly, and fibromuscular dysplasia in younger patients.

Endocrine excesses causing hypertension include:

Cortisol	• Cushing's disease/syndrome, adrenal tumours
Aldosterone	• Conn's syndrome — often associated with low potassium and metabolic alkalosis
Thyroxine	• hyperthyroidism
Catecholamine	• phaeochromocytoma
Growth hormone	• acromegaly.

Drugs — especially the oral contraceptive pill (OCP).

Remember: OCP + obesity + alcohol → elevated BP.

Others
- corticosteroids, that is, Prednisolone
- non-steroidal anti-inflammatory drugs (NSAIDs)
- cyclosporine commonly used for immunosupression in transplant recipients.

Others — hypertension is also a feature of vasculitis (e.g., systemic sclerosis and systemic lupus erythematosus — SLE) and coarctation of the aorta (see below).

With these in mind, begin your focused history.

4.9.3 *History*

Most patients with high blood pressure have no symptoms at all. Remember — elevated BP readings are often found incidentally, that is, during routine health checks in general practice or in clinics. So always remember to check the blood pressure!

Ask about:

Other ***risk factors*** for cardiovascular disease — see history and examination. Remember — these risk factors act synergistically to increase the patient's overall risk, and therefore the likely benefits from treatment.

- Smoking
- Diabetes mellitus
- Hypercholesterolaemia
- Family history of myocardial infarction

With hypertension, there is acceleration of atherosclerosis within the brain, coronary arteries, peripheral arteries and kidneys. With time, uncontrolled high blood pressure will cause target or end organ damage within these organs. Left ventricular hypertrophy can also develop as the heart is working harder to expel blood against an elevated blood pressure. Over time, this can limit diastolic filling and stroke volume and so lead to a form of heart failure.

4.9.4 *Complications from uncontrolled hypertension*

These can present as symptoms of **target organ damage**. These include:

- **Brain** (stroke or transient ischaemic attack) — especially in the presence of weak cerebral arteries as in Berry's aneurysm.
- **Heart** (left ventricular hypertrophy [LVH] or failure) — worsening exercise tolerance, ankle swelling, breathlessness-at-rest, angina, myocardial infarction, orthopnoea, and paroxysmal nocturnal dyspnoea [PND] — see heart failure).
- **Kidney** (renal impairment) — symptoms of uraemia, or frothy urine of proteinuria (both rare at the time of new diagnosis of hypertension).

- **Peripheral arterial disease**
  Ask about claudication: cramp-like pain or weakness at the back of the calves/thighs/buttocks on walking, relieved by rest.

'Claudication' originates from the Roman Emperor Claudius who walked with a limp. In Latin, 'claudicare' means 'to limp'.

4.9.5 *On examination*

The hypertensive patient needs a full cardiovascular examination — see the chapter on bedside examination. However, look carefully for ***signs*** of target/end organ damage.

- Heart — palpate for a sustained apical impulse/heave which may indicate left ventricular hypertrophy (LVH). Raised jugular venous pressure (JVP) and ankle swelling should prompt a search for other features of heart failure.
- Brain — offer to examine the central nervous system looking for evidence of focal neurology, e.g., hemiparesis secondary to a previous stroke.

If hypertension is severe or advancing rapidly, make sure you do *fundoscopy* to look for blurring of the optic disc margins, signifying papilloedema. The presence of papilloedema is a strong indicator of serious end-organ damage (which may include not only the eyes, but also the **brain**, **lungs** and **kidneys**). This is called **malignant hypertension** and its presence necessitates emergency admission to hospital for urgent treatment.

Although no specific cause is found in 90% of hypertensive patients, the 5% with specific **secondary causes** often present to medical exams. Don't be caught unprepared, get into the habit of looking for specific causes — look for features suggestive of **RED** (see below).

Renal

- Chronic renal failure — increase 'yellowish' pigmentation, arm — AV fistulae for dialysis, oedema.
- Adult polycystic kidney disease — abdominal mass in the flank.

- Renal artery stenosis — listen (2.5 cm above and lateral to the umbilicus) for a bruit — murmur due to turbulent flow from the stenosed renal arteries.

Endocrine/Drugs

- Cushing's syndrome/disease — moon face, central obesity, muscle wasting, and 'lemon-on-a-stick cushingoid-appearance', which may also be secondary to drugs such as corticosteroids.
- Phaeochromocytoma — sweating, tremor, paroxysmal hypertension and postural hypotension. If this is suspected, then screen for multiple endocrine neoplasia (MEN) type II (see appendix).

Others

- *Coarctation of the aorta* — a congenital narrowing in the aorta which is usually diagnosed in youth or early adulthood. This causes:
  - high pressure in the right arm
  - weak or absent pulses in the femoral arteries and legs (although these can easily be caused by atherosclerotic disease of the aorta or iliac)
  - radiofemoral delay between the right radial pulse and the femoral arteries (if the femorals are palpable). Blood pressure in the left arm may be similar to the right arm (if the coarctation is distal to the left subclavian) or much lower than the left arm (if the coarctation is proximal to the left subclavian).

Having examined the patient, the next step is to request investigations in order to localise your findings and determine the exact cause or exclude secondary causes of hypertension.

4.9.6 *Investigations in hypertension*

Always start with the simple things first:

- Blood test
  - Urea and electrolytes — abnormally high levels (particularly raised creatinine) may suggest renal impairment — this can

be the cause or a complication of hypertension. *Note*: Hypokalaemia may be a feature of treatment with diuretics, Conn's syndrome, or Cushing's disease.
  - o Fasting-lipid profile and blood glucose (screen for risk factors for cardiovascular disease).

- ➢ Urine dipstick — look for proteinuria and haematuria seen in glomerulonephritis.
- ➢ ECG — look for signs of left ventricular hypertrophy (see chapter on *Investigations — ECG interpretation*), and Q wave (indicative of previous myocardial infarction).
- ➢ Chest radiograph — cardiomegaly or features of heart failure. Rarely — inferior rib notching, suggestive of coarctation of the aorta. (In the first instance, radio-femoral delay, unequal arm pulses, weak or absent lower limb pulses, or systolic murmur, may trigger you to do a CT of the thoracic aorta to detect this rare condition.)

SPECIFIC TESTS

- Phaeochromocytoma — request urinary metanephrine, free catecholamines, and Vinyl Mandelic Acid (VMA).
- Renal disease — obtain mid-stream urine and sends for cells, casts, and protein present in glomerulonephritis, vasculitis or renal tumours.
- Cushing's disease/syndrome — urinary free cortisol, but don't forget to request a Dexamethasone suppression test (much more definitive).
- Thyroid disease — request a thyroid function test.

4.9.7 *How to measure blood pressure*

For a step-by-step guide, see the appendix. Note: Do not treat on the basis of an isolated reading alone, unless there is evidence of end-organ damage. Ideally, the diagnosis should be confirmed by an elevated blood pressure on three separate occasions.

4.9.8 *Management of the hypertensive patient*

Management consist of two broad interventions:

Non-pharmacological and **Pharmacological intervention**

Lifestyle interventions
- Stop smoking
- Lose weight
- Aerobic exercise
- Dietary (*DASH diet)
  - Increase consumption of fruits and vegetables
  - Reduce total fat and saturated fat intake, and salt intake.

Clinical Trials you ought to know:

ASCOT (**A** & **C** versus **B** & **D**)
- 19,000 patients

Combination of A & C reduced risk of stroke by 25%, MI by 15% and new-onset diabetes by 30%. Initiation of Atorvastatin significantly improved cardiovascular benefits compared with placebo.

HAPPHY (**B** versus **D**)
- 3,569 patients

The incidence of fatal stroke tended to be lower in the B than D group. Total mortality and total number of end-points were similar in both groups.

ALLHAT (compares **A** & **C** to **D**)
-33,357 patients

No significant difference in the reduction of risk of heart failure between A, C, & D. Forty per cent of patients required >1 drug to reach target BP.

ACD algorithm

A - Angiotensin Converting Enzyme ACE Inhibitor (*Ramipril*)
  - Angiotensin Receptor Blocker (*Irbesartan*)

B - Beta-blocker

C - Calcium channel Blocker (*Amlodipine*)

D - Diuretics

	Age <55 years	**Age >55 years or Black patients at any age**
Stage 1	**A**	**C or D**
Stage 2	**+ C/D**	or **C/D + A**
Stage 3	**A + C + D**	

Add:
- Further Diuretic therapy (D)
- Alpha-blocker, or
- Beta-blocker

Consider seeking specialist advice

*Dietary Approaches to Stop Hypertension diet – see Appendix

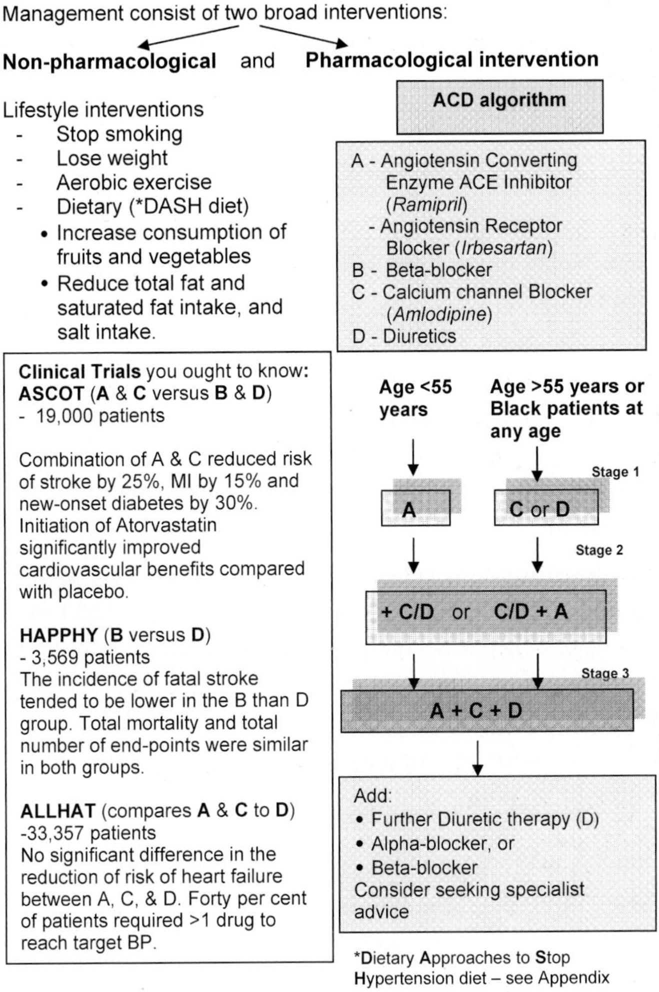

Figure 4.6 Management of the hypertensive patient

In order to address ***other risk factors*** for cardiovascular disease, patients also benefit from the addition of:

- ➢ Aspirin +/–
- ➢ Lipid lowering agent, e.g., statin.

ACE inhibitors are particularly useful in **diabetes** because they reduce microalbuminuria and retard the development of diabetic nephropathy. Alpha-blockers are useful in reducing male lower urinary tract symptoms — especially in **benign prostatic hyperplasia**.

Treatment targets

Therapeutic targets for blood pressure control:

<140/80 mmHg in the non-diabetic patient.
<125/75 mmHg in the patient with diabetes, renal impairment +/– established CVD.

To Impress!

What is the role of beta-blockers in the management of hypertension?

For decades, it was only beta-blockers and thiazide diuretics that had large-scale proof of efficacy in preventing strokes, heart attacks and deaths from hypertension. However, comparative trials in recent years have led to beta-blockers no longer being recommended as first-line agents in isolated hypertension. Their clinical benefit (especially in stroke prevention) is less good than **A, C** and **D**.

However they are still useful in:

i) patients with intolerance/contra-indications to ACE-inhibitors/ Angiotensin Receptor Antagonists,
ii) women of child-bearing potential (labetalol can be carried on during pregnancy), and
iii) patients with hypertension complicated by myocardial infarction, angina, fast atrial fibrillation, or heart failure.

4.10 Heart Failure

There are so many possible definitions of heart failure, and they may appear vague, so you can easily end up 'freezing' when asked for a definition.

A good basic definition is:

"Heart failure is the inability of the heart, usually because of disease of the **left ventricle**, to pump sufficient **cardiac output** to serve the **needs of the body** at a **normal filling pressure**".

Remember that when sitting still, most patients with heart failure have cardiac output in the normal range. What is **abnormal** is that they cannot raise this cardiac output to a 'normal' degree on exercise, and/or they have to have a high filling pressure to achieve a normal resting cardiac output.

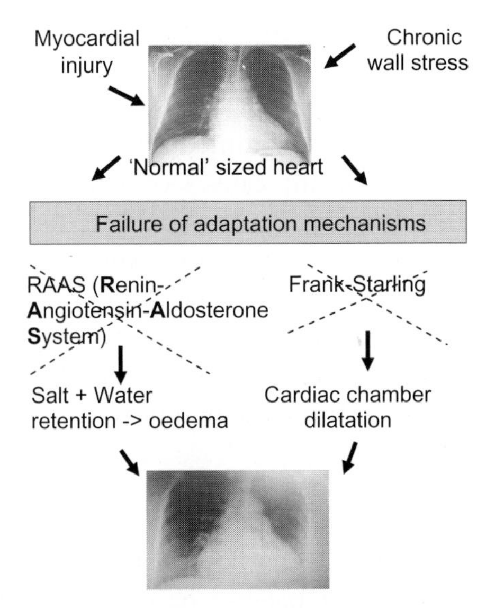

Figure 4.7 Pathophysiology of heart failure

Adaptive response **(Frank-Starling) explained**

Normally, increased wall strength will increase the *end diastolic return/volume* thus enhancing the preload. With more *preload,* the *stroke volume, and cardiac output* will also increase resulting in *myocardial hypertrophy* (increase in the size of the cell).

With time the size of the myocardium reaches a plateau and the chambers respond to further increases in wall stress by *dilatation* rather than hypertrophy. Thus there is **failure of adaptive response**.

Results in a 'failing', enlarged heart (cardiomegaly).

4.10.1 *What are the causes of heart failure?*

Heart failure is one of those conditions with an almost endless list of causes! You do not need to remember them all. To make it easier, we have broken down the list into simpler categories starting with the commonest (*you can also apply this method to other 'exhaustive lists'*). In the panic of an exam, knowing the common causes may still allow you to pass with high marks!

Commonest causes:

- **Coronary artery disease** (usually previous myocardial infarctions, but sometimes without)
- Unknown cause ('**Idiopathic** dilated cardiomyopathy')
- **Valvular disease**

Heart valve disease — most commonly regurgitant disease (mitral and aortic, for the clinically most important causes of left heart failure). Aortic stenosis may eventually cause heart failure, although untreated most such patients die of the other complications first.

The cardiomyopathies: Dilated CM, Restrictive CM, Hypertrophic CM

Less common:

Heart muscle disease — Cardiomyopathies (DCM >RCM >HCM) or viral myocarditis (behaves like DCM, but patients have raised inflammatory markers and a chance of complete resolution).

Toxins/Drugs — Alcohol and certain cancer chemotherapy drugs notoriously: Daunorubicin, Adramycin, 5-FU, and Herceptin (Trastuzumab) used for the treatment of metastatic breast cancer.

Rare causes:

Heart rhythm disease 'arrhythmias': Rarely, persistent tachycardia can lead to a weakening of the heart muscle, and thus heart failure.

Infiltrative: Amyloidosis, sarcoidosis (these are effectively a specific cause of RCM).

Metabolic/endocrine: Rarely, uncontrolled thyrotoxicosis, myxoedema or acromegaly can cause this.

Very rare causes in the developed world:

Nutritional: Beri-beri (Thiamine/Vitamin B1 deficiency), Kwashiorkor.

Inherited: Muscular dystrophies, such as, Duchene or Freidreich's ataxia.

Patients with 'chronic' heart failure are fairly common in hospitals, so your examination and knowledge of the subject must be slick!

4.10.2 *History*

Read in conjunction with the *Dyspnoea* section. Specific symptoms to elicit include:

- SOB — establish the triggers (exertion or rest)
- Orthopnoea
- Paroxysmal nocturnal dyspnoea
- Ankle swelling
- Decreasing exercise tolerance

Although less specific, patients may also complain of fatigue and palpitations.

4.10.3 *Examination*

Look out for the following **signs**:

- Pulse — tachycardia or pulsus alternans — (alternating weak and strong pulse — commonly quoted in books but is uncommon in practice).
- Neck — raised JVP (see Chapter 2 — *Bedside teaching* for full details).

- Chest (anteriorly) — laterally displaced apex beat secondary to cardiomegaly, right ventricular heave, gallop rhythm secondary to summation of heart sounds 3 (S3) + 4 (S4).
- Chest (posteriorly) — bibasal crackles suggest 'acute pulmonary oedema', stony dull percussion notes (heard in pleural effusion, also associated with reduced air entry).
- Abdomen — ascites (demonstrate shifting dullness/fluid thrill — see *Appendix*), hepatomegaly, pulsatile liver (seen in tricuspid regurgitation).
- Sacrum/legs — demonstrate 'pitting oedema' as previously described.

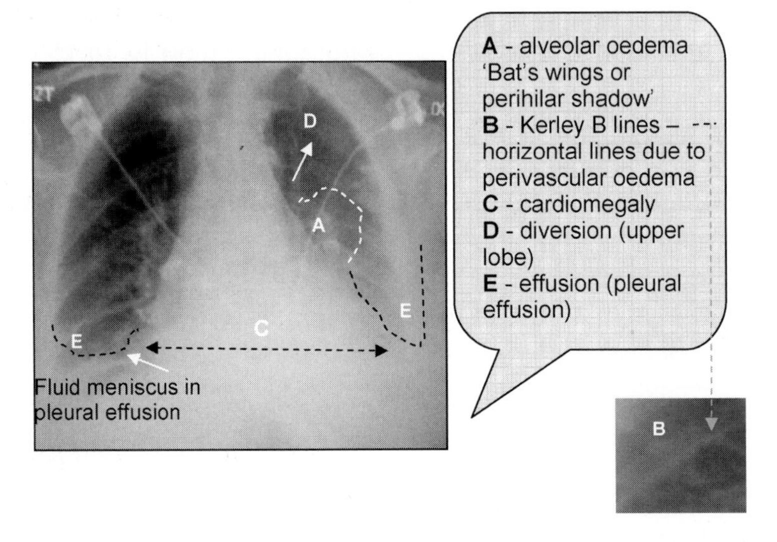

Figure 4.8 Radiological features of acute pulmonary oedema

4.10.4 *Investigations*

➢ Blood tests — full blood count (anaemia can mimic symptoms of heart failure); liver function tests — these may be deranged in hepatic congestion 'nutmeg liver'; urea and electrolytes — look for co-existing renal impairment.

Others: glucose and lipid profile (IHD), and thyroid function.

➢ Chest radiograph — see above.

- ECG — left ventricular hypertrophy may be seen in hypertension/aortic stenosis. Look for ischaemic changes — post-myocardial infarction (MI), especially an inferior MI.
- Echocardiography — **essential in all patients with heart failure!** Features include: ventricular hypertrophy, reduced ejection fraction (EF), valvular stenosis or regurgitation, hypokinesia/akinesia (may be secondary to previous MI or coronary artery disease).
- Cardiac catheterisation/angiography looking for ischaemia.
- Brain Natriuretic Peptide (BNP) — raised in heart failure (LV systolic dysfunction), associated with increase mortality. In environments where echocardiography is not routinely available, BNP can be used to screen patients: a low value makes heart failure very unlikely and can save the patient a trip to have echocardiography. Where echocardiography is routinely available, BNP may still have uses in monitoring the severity of the heart failure syndrome in the patient over time. Currently the cost of the assay has prevented it becoming universally used for diagnosis and monitoring.

4.10.5 *Further investigations in heart failure*

The following are useful in the assessment of cardiac function:

- Ambulatory ECG
- Exercise ECG
- Stress echo/multi gated acquisition scan (MUGA scan)

} See Chapter 3 *Investigations*

4.10.6 *Management of heart failure*

Initial management

- Sit patient upright.
- Start the patient on oxygen (that is, 10L/min for most, or 24–28% if the patient is CO_2-insensitive, has high CO_2 with COPD and ventilation is dependent on the hypoxic drive).
- Diuretics: 40–80 mg Frusemide (iv) stat.
- Opiate analgesia (Morphine 5–10 mg iv) plus antiemetic, that is, Metoclopramide (10 mg iv/po/im).

➢ Consider GTN/Frusemide infusion if symptoms persist in spite of the above measures (follow local hospital protocol).

The immediate management aims to **relieve** the initial symptoms, so it should be followed by measures that actually **reduce the morbidity and mortality** associated with heart failure. Follow the **5-step plan** (outlined in the diagram below — based on the NICE guideline for the management of chronic heart failure).

Further management — includes treating the underlying cause and **lifestyle modifications:**

- Fluid +/− salt restriction
- Smoking cessation and moderate alcohol intake
- Vaccination — annual influenza vaccine
- Weight loss (obesity increases heart workload)
- Exercise training (reduces mortality).

Five-step plan to reducing morbidity and mortality in heart failure

Step 1: Refer patients to a heart failure nurse for cardiac rehabilitation.

Step 2: Start **ACE-I/ ARA**. (Angiotensin Receptor Antagonist if ACE inhibitor not tolerated, that is, due to severe cough.)

Step 3: Add **beta-blocker** and titrate upwards (caution: it may worsen pulmonary oedema in acute situations).

Step 4: If the patient is still symptomatic despite the above steps add — **spironolactone or eplerenone** (indicated post-myocardial infarction).

See the drug section for contra-indications and monitoring of heart failure drugs.

Monitor treatment via:

- Daily weight (very useful marker of diuresis).
- Input/output chart (if the weight chart is not progressing as hoped). Aim for a negative fluid balance.
- Fluid restriction, for example, 1.5L per day.

Drugs that **relieve the symptoms** of heart failure:

Step 5: Seek specialist intervention.

- Diuretics — first line agent.
- Digoxin — (worsening or severe heart failure despite diuretics, ACE inhibitor/angiotensin receptor antagonist, beta-blocker therapy or when in atrial fibrillation).

To Impress!

Digoxin in heart failure:

The RADIANCE trial suggests that stopping Digoxin increases symptoms, whilst in the DIG-1 trial, starting Digoxin made no difference to mortality but reduced symptoms.

Loop diuretics in heart failure:

Loop diuretics (such as, Frusemide) are the drug-of-choice for reduction of fluid overload, and thus symptom relief. Discontinuation is likely to result in increased hospitalisation and mortality, yet there has been no formal clinical trial to demonstrate this!

Eplerenone: Aldosterone receptor antagonist (similar to spironolactone). Indication: reduction in cardiovascular death in patients with heart failure or LV systolic dysfunction following a myocardial infarction. Can cause hyperkalaemia — so monitor potassium.

Below is a summary of the evidence in support of the key drugs used in the management of heart failure.

Table 4.6 Management of heart failure — key trials and drugs

Drug	**Effect on mortality** in heart failure	**Clinical trials** supporting use in heart failure
ACE inhibitors	↓↓	CONSENSUS
Angiotensin receptor antagonists	↔	ELITE

(*Continued*)

Table 4.6 (*Continued*)

Drug	**Effect on mortality** in heart failure	**Clinical trials** supporting use in heart failure
Beta-blockers	↓↓↓	MERIT
Aldosterone antagonist — Spironolactone Eplerenone	↓↓↓	RALES
Digoxin	↔	RADIANCE DIG-1

4.11 Cardiac Resynchronisation Therapy (CRT)

A subgroup of heart failure patients with low ejection fractions have either prolonged atrio-ventricular (AV) delay or marked mistiming between the contraction of the left and right ventricles, or between the walls of the left ventricle. This is picked up from the ECG: left bundle branch block, together with an ejection fraction of <35%, seems to identify a group of patients many of whom benefit in terms of symptoms and survival from having CRT. (Studies are ongoing to see if detecting the mismatched contraction timing by echo or other imaging methods can help identify the right patients more precisely.)

4.11.1 *What is CRT?*

CRT or cardiac re-synchronisation therapy is an adjunct to drug therapy for **advanced** heart failure. CRT aims to shorten AV delay, reduce interventricular delay and decrease the event of symptomatic bradycardia which may present secondary to dys-synchrony in the contraction of both the left and right ventricles.

4.11.2 *How is re-synchronisation achieved?*

A biventricular (atrio-biventricular pacemaker) is implanted into the patient. Unlike a traditional pacemaker (see '4.15 Cardiac pacing') it has three leads: the usual two leads (atrial and ventricular leads) of a permanent pacemaker, plus a **third lead** which runs in the coronary sinus onto the free wall of the left ventricle. After atrial contraction, both ventricles are paced to contract at the same time, causing the heart to contract in a more efficient manner, resulting in improved cardiac function.

4.11.3 *Procedure*

As for permanent pacemaker — see *4.18 Cardiac pacing*.

4.11.4 *CRT-D versus CRT-P*

CRT can be done with or without an ICD (see 'implantable cardiac defibrillator'). An ICD can defibrillate or 'shock' the patient in the event of life-threatening arrhythmias (such as, ventricular tachycardia), but adds hugely to the cost. CRT-D is cardiac resynchronisation therapy with a defibrillator, whilst CRT-P includes a pacemaker.

4.11.5 *Complications*

These are generally rare. Thirty day operative mortality is <1% with a 5–10% failure rate. For other complications, see 'cardiac pacing' below.

4.11.6 *Evidence for its use*

- **In Sync Trial** (Gras *et al.*, 2002).
- **PAVE study** (see abbreviations) improved left ventricular ejection fraction (LVEF) and exercise test compared to right-ventricular paced patients. PAVE study has shown improved cardiac function (LVEF) and exercise tolerance (6 minute walk test) in CRT paced patients compared with right ventricular paced patients with class IV heart failure.
- **CARE-HF study** (2005), a large RCT of CRT-pacing, also demonstrates that CRT without ICD produces a substantial

absolute risk reduction of death and reduction in hospitalisation for heart failure, and improved quality of life.

To Impress!

NICE recommendations:

The UK's NICE Heart Failure Guideline of May 2007 recommends that resynchronisation therapy should be considered for patients with **moderate to severe symptoms of heart failure** (NYHA class 3 or 4), **left ventricular dysfunction with ejection fraction <35%, optimum drug therapy and regular pulse with evidence of abnormal electrical activity on ECG.**

4.12 Cardiomyopathy (CM)

The cardiomyopathies are a group of disorders resulting in diseased heart muscle. The WHO classification refers to four primary conditions:

- **Dilated** cardiomyopathy (**DCM**) — the commonest, by far!
- **Hypertrophic** cardiomyopathy (**HCM**)
- **Restrictive** cardiomyopathy (**RCM**)
- **Arrhythmogenic right ventricular** cardiomyopathy (**ARVC**).

4.12.1 *What are the causes of cardiomyopathy?*

Cause of cardiomyopathy can be inherited or acquired (see Fig. 4.9 on the following page). The figure below illustrates these.

4.13 Dilated Cardiomyopathy (DCM)

This is by far **the commonest cardiomyopathy**. In DCM the heart is often flabby and globular with a thin walled, large cavity left ventricle. With time, both ventricles progressively dilate (left ventricle > right ventricle), cardiac output is reduced and heart failure ensues.

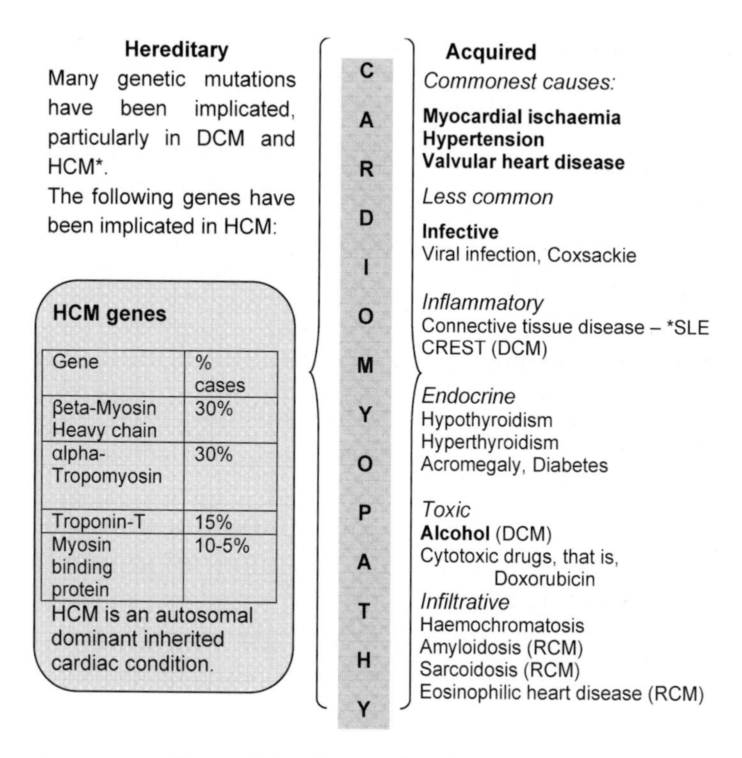

Figure 4.9 Causes of cardiomyopathy

*SLE — systemic lupus erythematosus.
CREST — calcinosis, Raynaud's, oEsophageal involvement, sclerodactyly, telangiectasia.

4.13.1 *History*

Ask about: symptoms of heart failure — breathlessness, fatigue reduced exercise tolerance, oedema, orthopnoea, and paroxysmal nocturnal dyspnoea (see 'heart failure').

Remember, the dilated flabby heart can also present as:

- Valve regurgitation — particularly mitral and tricuspid.
- Emboli — systemic/pulmonary (PE) with mural thrombus in the ventricles.
- Atrial fibrillation (AF) — especially in DCM secondary to alcohol.
- Syncope or sudden death.

4.13.2 *Examination*

Look for **signs** of heart failure with:

- hypotension
- small volume pulse/AF
- pan systolic murmur of mitral/ tricuspid regurgitation.

Reversible causes

These include:

- Ischaemic heart disease
- Valvular heart disease

Consider revascularisation in these patients.

4.13.3 *Investigations*

- ➢ Blood — full blood count (low haemoglobin), liver function test (alcohol excess), urea and electrolytes, viral serology, thyroid function (atrial fibrillation).
- ➢ Chest radiograph — cardiomegaly +/− features of heart failure.
- ➢ ECG — sinus tachycardia, atrial fibrillation, left ventricular (LV) hypertrophy.
- ➢ Echocardiography — large left and right ventricle, low ejection fraction (EF), poor movement of the posterior and septal wall. The dilated ventricles are prone to thrombus formation.
- ➢ Cardiac catheterisation — used to exclude coronary artery disease, which is a common cause of dilated left ventricle.

4.13.4 *Management of dilated cardiomyopathy*

Treatment focuses on two main factors:

i) symptom relief
ii) improving the prognosis

Medical treatment

These patients are treated for heart failure (see management of heart failure).

Cardiac transplant

In general, cardiac transplant is available to any patient with cardiomyopathy. However, in practice, transplantation is disproportionately often done on patients with dilated cardiomyopathy. This is because these patients are more likely to be young and less likely to have severe disease of other organs that would otherwise be a contra-indication (see 'To Impress' 4.13.5).

To Impress!

The dilated cardiomyopathy screen

If you suspect dilated cardiomyopathy then consider requesting the following additional investigations as part of the cardiomyopathy screen:

- Viral serology (Coxsackie, cytomegalovirus/Epstein Barr virus, HIV)
- Thyroid function test (?atrial fibrillation)
- Serum ferritin, iron and transferrin (haemochromatosis)
- Infective screen (HIV, Hepatitis C)

4.14 Hypertrophic Cardiomyopathy (HCM)

Most patients with HCM remain asymptomatic throughout life. In fact, hypertrophic cardiomyopathy is the **commonest cause of sudden cardiac death in children and young people**.

4.14.1 *History*

Focus on symptoms of **left ventricular outflow obstruction:**

- ➢ Angina
- ➢ Syncope or pre-syncopal episodes
- ➢ Breathlessness
- ➢ Palpitations due to arrhythmias
- ➢ **Family history of sudden death!**

4.14.2 *Examination*

Look for the following classical signs:

- Jerky carotid pulsation (generally only in severe cases).
- JVP: large 'a' wave (due to right ventricular flow obstruction).

- Double apical impulse (due to forceful atrial contraction against a non-complaint left ventricle → fourth heart sound).
- Ejection systolic murmur — loudest at the apex and left sternal edge (with no carotid radiation), but increases with a decrease in preload (Valsalva manoeuvre, standing) and is decreased by an increase in preload (squatting).
- Pansystolic murmur (of mitral regurgitation due to systolic anterior motion (SAM) — see below).

4.14.3 *Investigations*

- ECG — look for features of increase left ventricular strain, e.g., hypertrophy and T wave inversion (see the 'ECG' section).
- Chest radiograph — sometimes left atrial enlargement 'double heart border' silhouette is visible.
- Echocardiography — often diagnostic with the characteristic **ASH** (asymmetrical septal hypertrophy) **+/–SAM** (systolic anterior motion of the anterior mitral valve leaflet which abuts the septum in systole thereby causing dynamic left ventricular outflow tract obstruction — characteristic of hypertrophic obstructive cardiomyopathy — **HOCM**).
- Cardiac catheterisation — used to determine degree of outflow obstruction.
- 24-hour tape/Holter — looking for arrhythmias, particularly ventricular tachycardia (commoner in this patient group).
- **Pedigree analysis** — may reveal autosomal dominant inheritance pattern.

Management

Medical

- Beta-blocker (improves survival) or rate limiting calcium blocker (for treatment of angina and breathlessness).
- Amiodarone (for arrhythmias, note: Digoxin is contra-indicated in patients with atrial fibrillation and hypertrophic cardiomyopathy).
- Screen family members.

Surgical

- Septal ablation/myomectomy.
- Implantable cardiac defibrillator (ICD) — for patients at high risk of sudden death.

4.15 Restrictive Cardiomyopathy (RCM)

In this subgroup of patients, the walls of the ventricles become stiff, thus resisting or 'restricting' cardiac filling. This forces blood back up into the lungs (resulting in pulmonary congestion), the veins of the neck (raised JVP), and liver (hepatic congestion 'nutmeg liver').

Restrictive cardiomyopathy can be idiopathic, but has rare associations with amyloidosis, sarcoidosis, iron storage disease (e.g., Haemochromatosis) and eosinophilic heart disease (e.g., Loeffler's endocarditis, and Endomyocardial fibrosis).

4.15.1 *History*

- Breathlessness
- Fatigue (reduced exercise tolerance)
- Ankle/leg swelling — pedal oedema
- Abdominal swelling — hepatomegaly, ascites (essentially features of 'heart failure')

In addition to the above, ask specifically about:

- Palpitations or syncope (may suggest arrhythmias)
- Embolic phenomenon — both systemic and pulmonary
- Sudden death!

4.15.2 *Examination*

Look for **signs** of heart failure; pay close attention to the following:

- **Freidreich's sign** (high JVP with diastolic collapse of neck veins, also seen in constrictive pericarditis)

Restrictive cardiomyopathy is often confused with constrictive pericarditis; however only the later is amenable surgery — **pericardiectomy**.

- **Kussmaul sign** (raised JVP on inspiration, also seen in cardiac tamponade).

4.15.3 *Investigations*

As for heart failure, including: bloods, Chest radiograph, ECG, echocardiography, catheterisation, +/-cardiac biopsy.

4.15.4 *Management*

Treatment is limited and similar to heart failure treatment; however it can also be **palliative**. Although medical therapy has limited value, the following drugs may be used **cautiously** to avoid decreasing ventricular filling pressure and cardiac output:

- Diuretic
- ACE inhibitor
- Anti-arrhythmics +/-anticoagulation.

Cardiac pacing or even transplantation can be considered in arrhythmia.

4.16 Arrhythmogenic Right Ventricular Cardiomyopathy (ARVC)

In this subset of patients with cardiomyopathy, the right ventricle is replaced by **fibrous scar and fatty tissue** making it susceptible to **ventricular arrhythmias** (particularly ventricular tachycardia, fibrillation or ectopic beats). The risk of risk of sudden death and bi-ventricular failure is thus increased in these patients.

Pattern of inheritance can be both autosomal dominant or autosomal recessive.

4.16.1 *History, examination and investigations*

As for dilated cardiomyopathy with the following additions:

- **ECG — Epsilon waves.** These are small deflections seen in the ST segment immediately after an S deflection. Best seen in V1 — V4 (in ~30% of patients). It is due to delayed excitation of myocytes of the right ventricle (as the RV consists of islands of viable myocytes surrounded by fibrofatty tissue). They are also seen in other diseases of the right heart, that is, right ventricular infarct and sarcoidosis.

- **Cardiac CT/MR** can be superior to echo in suspected ARVC.
- **Endomyocardial biopsy** (although a negative biopsy does not exclude ARVC as viable myocardium may be surrounded by fibrofatty tissue).

4.16.2 *Management of arrhythmogenic right ventricular cardiomyopathy*

Medical:

Treatment includes anti-arrhythmic drugs, although an implantable cardiac defibrillator (ICD) may be preferable in cases of serious arrhythmias.

Surgical:

Heart transplant should also be considered.

To Impress!

What is the role of **heart transplant** in cardiomyopathy?

Heart transplants offer hope of long-term survival for patients in whom medical treatment has failed. Five year survival is ~65%. Only about 400 heart transplants/annum in the UK, due to organ shortage.

Indication: Cardiomyopathy-dilated (DCM), restrictive (RCM), hypertrophic (HCM), and arrhythmogenic right ventricular cardiomyopathy (ARVC).

Contra-indications: Poor renal function, liver failure, advance age (usually >60 yrs), severe pulmonary hypertension.

Signs of rejection: These include malaise, low-grade fever, arrhythmias, and features of heart failure.

> *Note*: **Heart-lung transplant** — as in patients with cystic fibrosis or Eisenmenger's syndrome (ES). ES = Left heart to Right heart shunt → pulmonary hypertension → reversal of shunt: Right to Left).

4.17 Implantable Cardiac Defibrillator (ICD)

The ICD (sometimes called the automated-ICD or AICD, and often referred to in speech as the 'defib') looks like a pacemaker, but is much more expensive and elaborate. It is a little bigger in size to allow for greater battery capacity, and can do everything a pacemaker can do. In addition, it can defibrillate or '**shock**' the patient in the event of a life-threatening arrhythmia, that is, ventricular tachycardia. **ICDs are superior to anti-arrhythmic drugs in reducing mortality in patients at increased risk of ventricular tachyarrhythmias.**

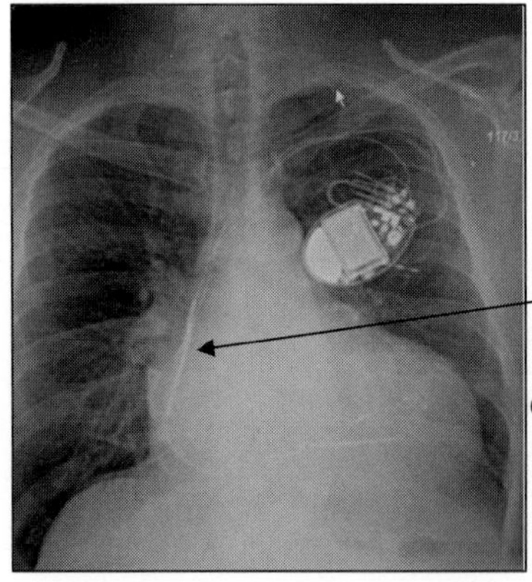

Figure 4.10 Chest radiograph showing a biventricular-ICD. Like a pacemaker, an ICD has a generator box, lead wires and electrodes at the tip of the lead wires (see 'cardiac pacing').

4.17.1 *Indication*

ICDs are implanted to treat ventricular tachycardia (VT) or ventricular fibrillation (VF). For other indications, see the table below.

Primary prevention	Secondary prevention
1. MI with ejection fraction (EF) <35% (NHYA class ≤ 3) 2. Familial heart disease associated with a high risk of death, that is: • Cardiomyopathy (see above) HCM > ARVC > DCM • Long QT syndrome • Brugada syndrome	No treatable cause *plus* • Cardiac arrest due to VT/VF • Spontaneous sustained VT → syncope/significant haemodynamic compromise See NICE guidelines www.nice.org

4.17.2 *How does an implantable cardiac defibrillator work?*

Modern ICDs do more than just immediately defibrillate. For ventricular tachycardia (VT), they first try a sequence of fast pacing algorithms that attempt to disrupt the regular VT cycle in order to restore sinus rhythm. These attempts are called Anti-Tachycardia Pacing (ATP). If these fail, or if the rhythm becomes VF or is VF from the outset, the ICD will move on to deliver an electric shock.

A shock from an ICD is typically 15–30 J, that is, an order of magnitude lower than what you give with an external defibrillator. It is effective because it is delivered directly to the heart.

4.17.3 *Procedure*

As for permanent pacemaker — see details on cardiac pacing (below).

4.17.4 *Follow-up*

Following implantation of the device, patients are followed-up for:

- Evaluation of device

- Interrogation (retrieval of stored information, e.g., events of ICD discharge)
- Replacement of battery/generator (usually every 3–5 years)
- Lead impedance testing (pacing impedance, shock impedance).

4.17.5 *Evidence for their use (see Chapter 9 'Abbreviation' for list of trials)*

Anti-arrhythmic drugs *versus* ICD for sustained VT/VF:

Primary prevention • MUSTT/MADIT	ICD is superior to anti-arrhythmic drugs in reducing ***mortality in patients at ↑ risk of VT.***
Secondary prevention • AVID/CID/CASH	ICDs also ***reduce mortality from sudden cardiac arrhythmias in survivors of VT/VF.***

4.18 Cardiac Pacing

Implantation of a cardiac pacing device can be the solution in patients with persistent or intermittent bradycardias, or those presenting with long pauses and delays in conduction between cardiac chambers.

A pacemaker is an electrical device, placed under the skin of the chest, with electrical leads (usually two), running through the subclavian vein, superior vena cava, and into the heart (usually right atrium and right ventricle).

The pacemaker detects natural electrical activity in the atrium and the ventricle. If the atrial activity is too slow, it delivers an electrical **stimulus to the atrium**. If the delay between atrial and ventricular activity is too long, it delivers a **stimulus to the ventricle**.

When the patient becomes physically active, the pacemaker detects this by sensing movement (with an accelerometer) or increased respiration (using **impedance** measurements across the chest). It accordingly increases the rate at which it expects the heart to beat, which may result in it pacing faster, or starting to pace when it was previously only observing.

If the patient goes into atrial fibrillation, the atrial electrical rate rises to many hundred beats per minute. It is important that the pacemaker detects this and does not try to pace the ventricle at a matching speed. Instead, it must 'switch modes' and become a purely ventricular pacemaker, pacing only when the ventricular rate falls too low. It quietly observes the atrium so that, when sinus rhythm returns, it can return to its previous function.

The behaviour described above is that of a '**DDDR** pacemaker', the most common form of pacemaker implanted (see table below).

Apart from the DDDR pacemaker, there are two other pacemakers that you are likely to come across.

The **VVIR** pacemaker which has no atrial lead is used for patients with permanent atrial fibrillation. It bypasses the atrium — sensing and pacing at the ventricules and is thus used in atrial fibrillation.

The atrio-biventricular (or 'biventricular' or 'Cardiac Resynchronisation Therapy' or '**CRT**') pacemaker is one that is placed not in order to speed up the heart, but as a special means of benefiting some patients with heart failure. Unlike the DDDR pacemaker, it has three leads (see CRT above).

At this point, let us review our own 'natural' cardiac pacing mechanism.

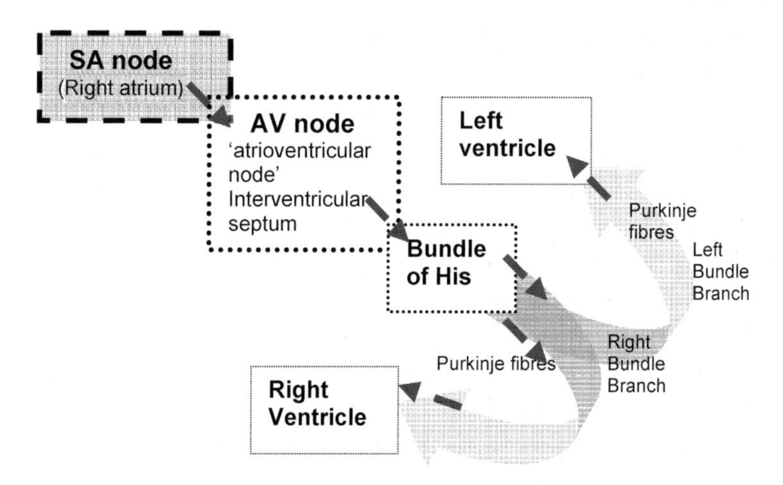

Figure 4.11 Conducting system of the heart

4.18.1 *DDDR, VVIR — what does it mean?*

Here is a guide to understanding the pacemaker language.

- Pacemakers can be: single or dual-chambered, or even biventricular.
- This terminology depends on the capacity of the pacing device to **sense** or **pace** in one or both chambers. So a dual chamber pacemaker has two pacing leads — one in the right atrium, and the other in the right ventricle enabling sensing and pacing from both chambers.

Table 4.7 Understanding pacing nomenclature

Chamber(s) paced	**Chamber(s)** sensed	**Response** to sensing	**Rate** modulation	Multisite pacing
O = None	O = None	O = None	O = None	O = None
A = Atrium	**A** = Atrium	**T** = Triggered	**R** = Rate modulation	A = Atrium
V = Ventricle	**V** = Ventricle	**I** = Inhibited		**V** = Ventricle
D = Dual (A+V)	**D** = Dual (A+V)	**D** = Dual (T+I)		**D** = Dual (A+V)

Using the table above, a **VVIR** pacemaker is:

Ventricle paced	**V**entricle sensed	**I**nhibition (response to pacing)	**R**ate responsive

In contrast, a **DDDR** pacemaker has:

Dual chamber pacing	**D**ual chamber sensing	**D**ual response to pacing — inhibition and trigger	**R**ate responsive

4.18.2 *What are the indications for pacing?*

Common indications:

- Symptomatic bradycardia
- Sinus node dysfunction
- Symptomatic heart block

} See Bradyarrhythmias

- Post-acute myocardial infarction (heart block)
- Neurocardiogenic syncope (reflex syncope)
- Pacing in special conditions, that is, hypertrophic cardiomyopathy, sleep apnoea
- Cardiac re-synchronisation therapy (see heart failure)

4.18.3 *Types of pacing*

Pacing can be:

- ➢ Transvenous (insertion of temporary pacing wires)
- ➢ Internal (permanent pacemaker)
- ➢ External (that is, with defibrillator pads in an emergency).

Transvenous pacing

This is an invasive technique that involves the insertion of a pacing lead/wire from the pacemaker generator (outside the body), into the right ventricle via a central venous catheter.

Temporary pacing is potentially life-saving and can be used in the following conditions:

- ➢ to correct profound bradycardia after an acute MI (particularly an inferior MI), or complete heart block
- ➢ whilst awaiting a permanent pacemaker
- ➢ when a temporary measure is indicated, that is, bradycardia secondary to drug overdose or Intensive Care Unit (ICU) patients after cardiac surgery.

Permanent pacing (permanent pacemaker — PPM)

The internal/permanent pace maker (PPM) consists of three parts:

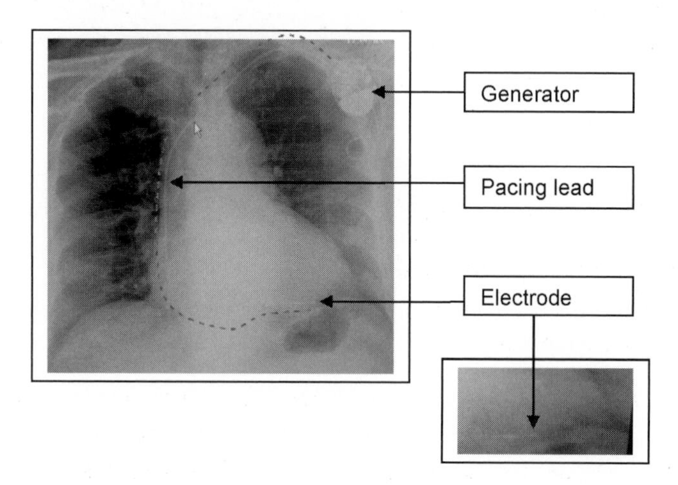

Figure 4.12 VVIR pacemaker. The dotted line traces the outline of the pacing lead.

Table 4.8 Components of a permanent pacemaker

Generator	• The 'artificial sinoatrial node' where impulses are generated to control the heart rate. • It is placed subcutaneously — palpable just below the left collarbone (typically). • Made of titanium, it is the size of a small match box. • It will last approximately 5–10 years.
Pacing Lead/s	• This is attached to the generator box. • It consists of one (as in a VVIR — above) or two platinum wires (as in DDDR — atrial and ventricular wires). • Pacing wires rest in the right atrium or right ventricle. • They carry impulse to the electrode.
Electrode	• This is found at the tip of the pacing lead/wire. • It is embedded into the heart muscle and delivers the necessary electrical impulse to the heart.

External pacing

In an **emergency**, there is often not even enough time to place a temporary pacing lead internally, or it may not be safe to do so. In such situations, it is possible to pace the heart externally through the chest, although some find it too uncomfortable to use for more than a brief time.

4.18.4 *How to use an external pacing device*

Step 1: Place two pacing pads onto the chest wall in the AP (anterior/posterior) or AL (anterior/lateral) position with the leads attached to a pacemaker.

Step 2: With the pads in place, select the pacing mode and pacing rate, whilst increasing the current gradually until 'electrical capture'. The pacemaker is said to be 'capturing' the heart rate when a pacing spike is seen in front of every QRS complex (below). Upon capture, re-assess the patient for clinical response — feel for a pulse with each QRS complex, check the blood pressure, and so on.

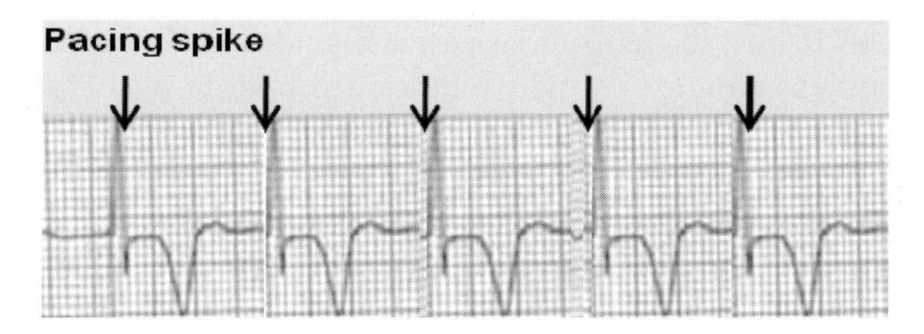

Figure 4.13 'Capture ECG' — showing a pacing spike before every QRS complex. Note: The QRS complexes are wide >120 milli-seconds.

4.18.5 *Insertion of a permanent pacemaker*

Before the 'Cath lab'

Internal pacing devices (that is, a permanent pacemaker) are inserted in the cardiac catheterisation laboratory ('Cath lab'). Before the 'Cath lab', ensure that the patient is adequately prepared:

- Take blood for full blood count, urea and creatinine, CRP and clotting screen
- Establish intravenous access
- Start prophylactic antibiotic cover to protect against skin infection (follow hospital protocol).

Procedure for the insertion

Insertion of the permanent pacing system is usually complete in approximately 1 hour.

- ➢ The area under the left clavicle is anaesthetised using local anaesthetic, that is, lignocaine.
- ➢ An incision is made below the clavicle (within this area).
- ➢ Pacing lead(s)/wire is inserted through the incision into a large vein (that is, the left subclavian), and guided under imaging to the right atrium +/− right ventricle (to both in dual chamber pacing) where the tip (with the electrode) is directly attached to the heart muscle.
- ➢ The proximal end of the lead/wire is then attached to the generator, which is then implanted subcutaneously or submuscularly below the clavicle.
- ➢ The incision is then closed with sutures.

Note: The function of the lead is usually tested before it is connected to the heart.

Pacemaker interrogation

This involves evaluating the pacing thresholds, lead impedance, and battery voltage. There is also a review of stored ECGs during subsequent out-patient follow-ups.

After the 'Cath lab' — on the ward

After testing the leads (to ensure that they are working), the patient is then transferred to the ward for cardiac monitoring (via telemetry). Be vigilant for displacement of the pacing lead as this commonly occurs within 24 hours of lead insertion. This may present as failure to capture (absence of pacing spikes on ECG).

Post-procedural checks

Post-procedural checks	Complications post-procedure
➢ Don't forget to request a **chest radiograph** post-procedure to check the position of the pacing leads, and to look for a pneumothorax. ➢ Ensure that the patient is on prophylactic antibiotics for a further five days or as per hospital protocol (see Investigations above).	Local • Haematoma, bleeding • Cellulitis • Pneumothorax • Pneumoperitoneum Systemic • Infective endocarditis Mechanical • Failure to output • Failure to capture • Over-sensing • Under-sensing *Pacemaker syndrome

*Symptoms of fullness in neck, pounding in the neck and head due to atrio-ventricular dys-synchrony.

Chapter 5

Cardiovascular Drugs

5.1 Antiplatelet Agents

5.1.1 *Aspirin*

Aspirin is used in cardiology for its antiplatelet properties, that is:

- Prevention of myocardial infarction (primary and secondary)
- Prevention of stroke in atrial fibrillation (AF)
- Prevention of death in acute coronary syndrome (ACS)

Primary Prevention:

34% reduction in MI

Secondary Prevention:

27% reduction in cardiovascular events

ACS:

35–50% reduction in cardiovascular events

Mechanism of action

Long-term use in low doses (typically 75 mg od) prevents **stroke** and **myocardial infarction**. It does this by irreversibly inhibiting the enzyme Cyclo-oxygenase (COX) thereby inhibiting the formation of thromboxane A2 in platelets and preventing platelet aggregation. There is convincing evidence of benefit in both primary and secondary prevention. Aspirin is also useful in **acute coronary syndromes**, and in the long-term management of patients with tissue **valve replacements** and **atrial fibrillation**.

Prescribing information

- Low dose 75 mg OD (once daily) for prevention

- High dose 300 mg (one-off dose for treatment of acute coronary syndrome/MI)

> **Key point:**
> Aspirin not only potentiates bleeding as a result of its antiplatelet properties but also **creates** new ulcers, by impeding gastric epithelial perfusion.

Main side effects

- ➢ Bleeding!
  - ~0.6% risk of gastro-intestinal haemorrhage (if patient is at high-risk, a **proton pump inhibitor** can be added). *Note*: Bleeding risk is dose dependent (CURE 2003).
- ➢ Bronchospasm — up to a-fifth of asthmatics can get this.
- ➢ Intracranial and extracranial haemorrhage.
- ➢ Can antagonise diuretics and cause fluid retention.

Contra-indications

- Children < 12 due to the risk of Reyes Syndrome*
- True allergic reaction
- Haemophilia and other bleeding disorders
- Peptic ulceration

> Determine whether it's a true allergy by asking about facial or laryngeal oedema or bronchospasm. Many patients wrongly classify 'dyspepsia' as allergy.

---

*Reyes Syndrome is a severe progressive encephalitic illness affecting children accompanied by fatty infiltration of the liver.

Evidence for its use

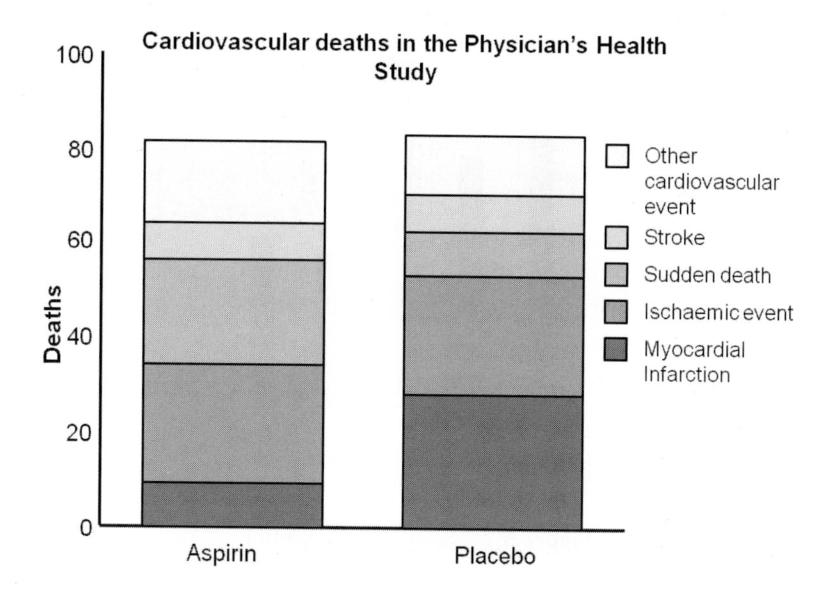

Figure 5.1 Primary prevention

Twenty two thousand and seventy-one American male physicians between 40 and 84 were randomised to aspirin or placebo. Results showed that aspirin reduced the risk of first myocardial infarction by 44% ($p < 0.00001$).

N Engl J Med 1989 Dec 28;321(26):1825–8.

In the event of surgery

Aspirin may need to be stopped five to seven days prior to surgery if there is a high risk of uncontrollable bleeding.

The dilemma — benefit versus harm?

The higher the baseline risks to the patient, the greater the expected reduction in death or myocardial infarction from having aspirin. But aspirin can also induce bleeding, intracranially and extracranially

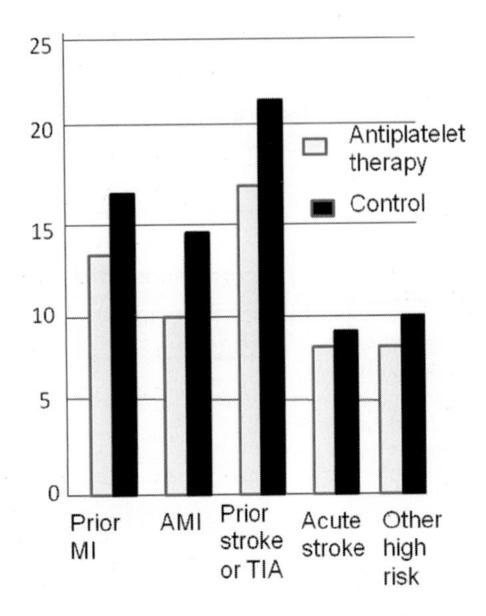

Figure 5.2 Secondary prevention

A meta-analysis of 237 studies including 135,000 patients comparing aspirin and a placebo. Reduction by 1/3rd of non-vascular event and reduction in non-fatal MI by 1/3rd. One-sixth reduction in vascular deaths.

Anti-thrombotic Trialists' Collaboration. Lancet 2002

(generally in the gut). Therefore the baseline risk of death and MI is important. The higher the baseline risk, the more likely it is to be worthwhile to take aspirin. For very low baseline risk, the harm from aspirin may exceed the benefit.

5.1.2 *Clopidogrel*

Clopidogrel (the first widely used agent of the thienopyridine class, which now also includes prasugrel) works by irreversibly blocking the ADP receptor (P2Y12) on platelet membranes and prevents platelet aggregation. In several settings, it is used as an adjunct, or alternative, to aspirin, in prevention of coronary or cerebral thrombosis.

Indications

- Secondary prevention of cardiovascular disease (CVD), as an adjunct or alternative to aspirin
- In acute coronary syndrome, as an adjunct to aspirin
- For patients undergoing coronary artery stenting, in combination with aspirin, for prevention of sudden stent thrombosis; duration of clopidogrel is usually longer for those receiving drug-eluting stents

In the event of surgery

In patients taking long-term clopidogrel, this is usually stopped at least one week beforehand. But if a patient has had recent coronary stenting, stopping clopidogrel risks coronary stent thrombosis, and specialist advice should be sought.

Prescribing information

- Loading dose 300 mg
- Maintenance dose 75 mg

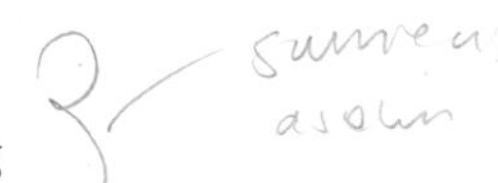

Side effects

- Bleeding (25% reduction in relative risk compared with aspirin)
- Gastrointestinal upset
- Bone marrow suppression

Contra-indications

- Active bleeding
- Breast feeding

Evidence for its use

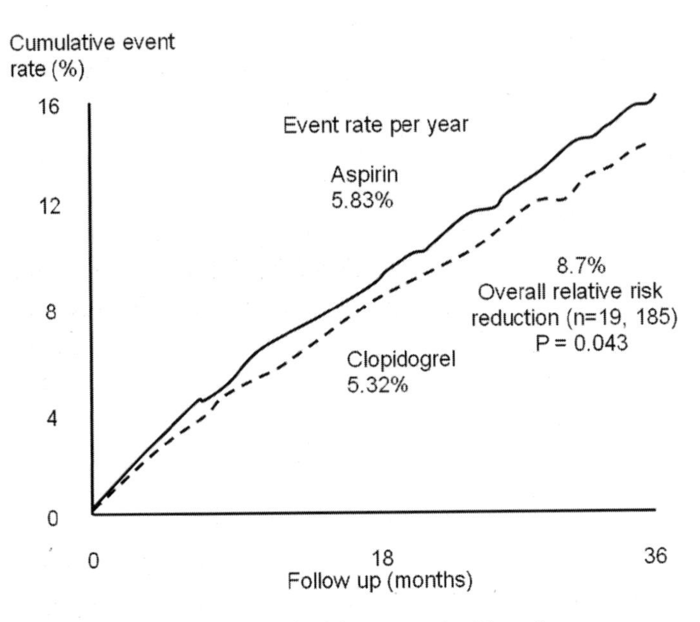

Figure 5.3 Aspirin versus clopidogrel

Although Clopidogrel may be marginally more effective in event prevention than aspirin, it is many times more expensive. Aspirin is generally recommended unless the patient has a specific intolerance.

CAPRIE Lancet 1996

5.1.3 *Dipyridamole*

This drug has multiple mechanisms, including prolonging the half-life of extracellular adenosine, and phosphodiesterase 5 inhibition. It inhibits platelets and causes vasodilatation. Its previous role as an adjunct to aspirin in coronary heart disease is largely now replaced by clopidogrel. It continues to be used as an adjunct (or alternative) to aspirin for stroke prevention (*European Stroke Prevention Study 2*). Because of its short half-life, it needs to be administered three times a day, or given as a proprietary long-acting once-daily preparation.

Side effects

- Gastrointestinal (GI) upset (most common!)
- Vasodilatation causing flushing, headache and tachycardia
- Bleeding, and thrombocytopenia (rare)

Adverse drug interactions

One of its mechanisms is the prolongation of the retention of adenosine in the extracellular space, by inhibiting its uptake into cells and inhibiting its breakdown. Therefore, be very careful if administering adenosine to a patient who is on dipyridamole: the bradycardia/asystole that results may be more severe and prolonged than you expect!

5.1.4 *Glycoprotein IIb/IIa receptor antagonists*

These inhibit the final common pathway of platelet aggregation by blocking the binding of fibrinogen to receptors on platelets. The most commonly used agents are:

- abciximab (*ReoPro*) Monoclonal antibody to GIIb/IIIa
- tirofiban } Non-peptide GIIb/IIIa antagonists
- eptifibatide }

Indications

They reduce cardiovascular events by 10% in patients with acute coronary syndrome. During percutaneous coronary intervention (PCI), this figure is increased by 20–30%. Long-term use of these agents in secondary prevention has been reported to increase mortality. Therefore they are only used as adjuvant (under specialist supervision) in patients with ACS undergoing, or waiting to undergo, primary/percutaneous coronary intervention (PCI).

Prescribing information

By intravenous infusion — varies according to local hospital protocol.

NICE recommendations (2005)

GIIb/IIIa inhibitors are recommended for use in the initial management of patients with unstable angina/NSTEMI in combination with aspirin and unfractionated heparin at **high risk** of myocardial infarction (MI) or sudden death.

Side effects:

- bleeding
- thrombocytopenia

Contra-indications:

- active internal bleeding
- major surgery
- breast feeding
- severe hypertension

5.2 Anticoagulants

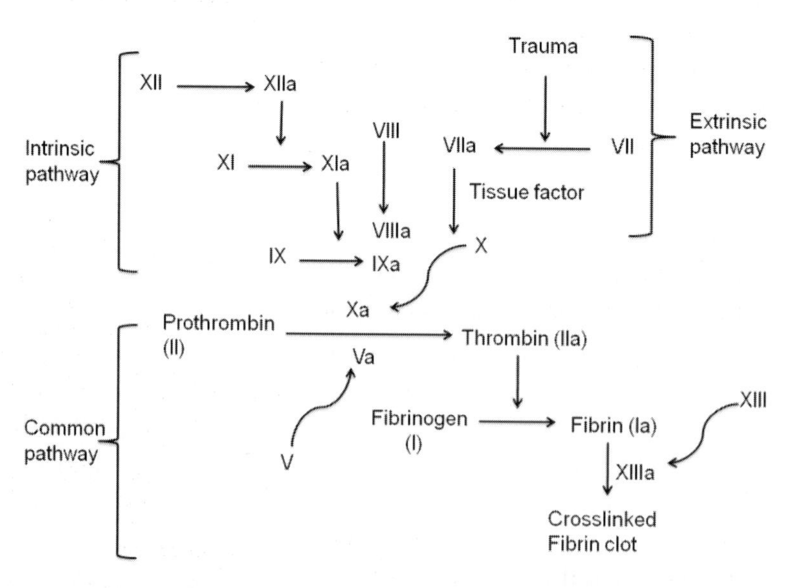

Figure 5.4 The diagram above illustrates the coagulation cascade

5.2.1 *Heparin*

Heparin is naturally produced by basophils and mast cells. Standard heparin works by binding to and activating antithrombin III, which then inactivates thrombin and other clotting factors, that is, factor Xa. It can be given intravenously or subcutaneously but is digested when ingested orally.

— **Fractionated low molecular weight heparin (LMWH)**

- for example, dalteparin (fragmin), enoxaparin (clexane)
- works by inhibiting factor Xa
- longer half-life
- given once/twice daily
- no need to monitor APTT

Caution in patients with a creatinine >300 as clexane undergoes renal excretion. In renal failure use UFH instead of LMWH.

— **Unfractionated heparin (UFH)**

- half-life of approximately 1 hour
- give by continuous infusion
- requires APTT monitoring 4 to 6 hours
- anticoagulant effects can be easily reversed

Indications

- Acute coronary syndrome
- Atrial fibrillation
- Deep vein thrombosis (DVT), pulmonary embolism (PE), and valve replacement

Prophylaxis

- General surgery in **'high risk'** patients — subcutaneous 5000 U 2 hours prior to surgery, then every 8–12 hours for 7 days

'**High risk**' patients
- obesity
- malignant disease
- history of DVT/PE
- over 40
- established thrombophilic disorder
- undergoing large/complicated procedures

Bear in mind other methods of reducing the risk of DVT including the use of thromboembolic deterrent stockings (TEDs) and pneumatic calf pumps during surgery.

Side effects

- bleeding (0–3%)
- hypersensitivity
- hyperkalaemia
- osteoporosis
- **H**eparin **I**nduced **T**hrombocytopenia — see **HIT** (opposite). Stop heparin immediately!

To Impress! — HIT

This usually occurs with a **fall in platelet count to <50% in days 5–10 of therapy**. Heparin-induced thrombocytopenia (HIT) can cause a paradoxical **risk of new thrombosis, both arterial and venous!** This is due to the formation of antibodies against platelet factor 4 (PF4). Stop heparin immediately, and consider an alternative anticoagulant, e.g., Lepuridin.

Contra-indications

- haemophilia
- thrombocytopenia
- peptic ulcer disease
- severe hypertension
- severe liver disease
- recent cerebral haemorrhage

In overdose

The effects of heparin can be reversed by ***protamine sulphate*** given as an intravenous injection over 10 minutes. One milligram neutralises 80–100 units of heparin when given within 15 minutes of heparin. Note: Protamine in excess has an anticoagulant effect.

5.2.2 *Warfarin*

Warfarin is a coumarin anticoagulant and works by inhibiting the synthesis of ***vitamin K dependent clotting factors***, that is, factor II, VII, IX and X as well as protein S and C. It is metabolised by the liver enzyme cytochrome P450 and therefore has many potential adverse drug interactions. It has a half-life of 48–72 hours, and is monitored via the ***INR*** (International Normalised Ratio).

Indications

- treatment of venous thromboembolism (VTE)
- and in cardiology it is used as VTE prophylaxis in:
  - Atrial fibrillation
  - Mechanical heart valves
  - Dilated cardiomyopathy/left ventricular aneurysm

Prescribing information

A typical starting regimen is usually 10 mg on the first day, then 5 mg on the second and third days (or as per hospital protocol). The desired INR will depend on the patient's underlying diagnosis. See section *Patients On Warfarin* in Chapter 2 *Bedside teaching* for more information.

Side effects

- haemorrhage
- transient hypercoaguable state
- alopecia, rash, skin necrosis
- teratogenicity

Contra-indications

- active bleeding
- dissecting aneurysm
- severe hypertension
- pregnancy
- liver or renal failure

Table 5.1 Drug interactions

Drugs that *increase* the effect of warfarin 'inhibitors'	Drugs that *decrease* the effect of warfarin 'inducers'
• Acute alcohol • Amiodarone • Antibiotics, that is: ➢ Cimetidine ➢ Omeprazole ➢ Simvastatin	• Phenytoin • Carbamazepine • Rifampicin • Oral contraceptive pill • Spironolactone • St. John's Wort

In the event of surgery

- ➢ stop three to five days prior to surgery and replace with heparin
- ➢ INR should be <1.2 for open surgery and <1.5 for open procedures (or as per local hospital protocol)

5.2.3 *Thrombolytics/Fibrinolytics*

Thrombolytics work by activating plasminogen to form plasmin which degrades fibrin and consequently breaks up the thrombi. Thrombolysis is **recommended early** or at least within 12 hours of presenting with symptoms of myocardial infarction in the absence of percutaneous coronary intervention (PCI).

Examples of thrombolytic agents

- streptokinase
- tissue plasminogen activator (tPA), reteplase, tenecteplase
- urokinase

Currently, in the absence of a Primary Coronary Intervention (PCI) unit, streptokinase is the cheapest alternative agent. However, once a patient has been treated with it, they form neutralising antibodies 4 days after administration and therefore require the slightly more expensive tPA or reteplase for subsequent reinfarctions.

Indications

When there is an urgent need to breakdown fibrin clot

- myocardial infarction (if emergency PCI is not available) — both streptokinase and alteplase have been shown to reduce absolute mortality by 1–2%.
  - ➢ streptokinase: 1.5 MU in 100 ml 5% dextrose/0.9% saline over 30–60 minutes
- life-threatening venous thrombosis/pulmonary embolus
- arterial thrombus
- stroke

Prescribing information

Fibronolytics should be given as early as possible after MI within 12-hours of a heart attack. 1,500,000 U over 60 minutes.

Allergic reactions are relatively common! Stopping and restarting infusion at a slower rate can reduce these effects.

Side effects

- bleeding (stroke, puncture sites, peptic)
- allergic reaction, hypotension, reperfusion arrhythmias

Contra-indications

- recent haemorrhage, trauma or surgery
- active bleeding
- recent stroke/transient ischaemic attack (TIA)
- active peptic ulceration, varices
- aortic dissection
- severe hypertension
- pregnancy

Treat each patient as an individual, carefully weighing the benefits of thrombolysis against the risk of bleeding!
Note: Risk of haemorrhagic stroke is 0.5–1%.

Evidence for their use

Fibrinolytic Therapist Trialists' Collaborative group showed the overall relative risk reduction in 35-day mortality with treatment is 18% (13% versus 8–9%).

UK National Service Framework

Advocates a door to needle time of <60 minutes.

Angiographic studies have shown tPA and reteplase to be more effective than streptokinase at opening coronary arteries (70% versus 35%). Although there is no evidence of a difference in 30-day mortality between the three drugs, some services use these agents preferentially, because their cost is no longer prohibitively high.

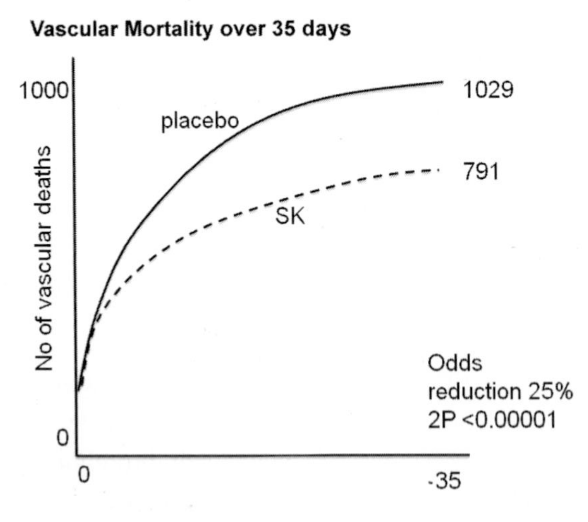

Figure 5.5 Benefits of reperfusion therapy in acute myocardial infarction

Multicenter, Multinational RCT of 17,187 patients with MI showed that streptokinase reduces all cause mortality when compared with placebo.

ISIS-2. Lancet 1988

50
40
30
20
10
0
Reduction in Mortality
47
23
17
10.6
< 1 hr
< 3 hrs
3-6 hrs
6-9 hrs
Hours following an MI

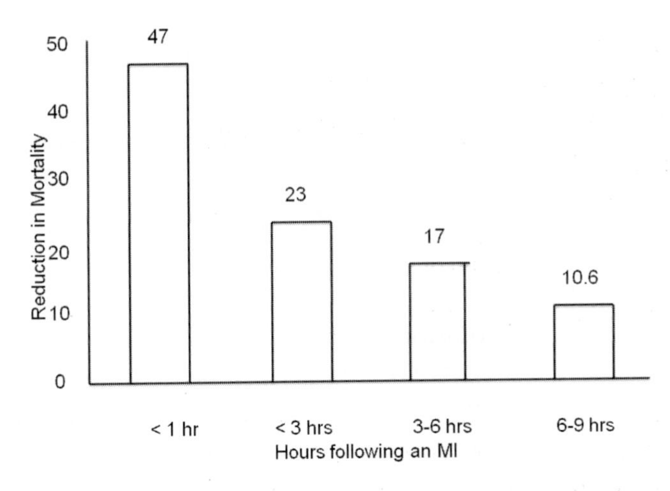

Figure 5.6 Benefits of early reperfusion in myocardial infarction

Eleven thousand eight hundred and six patients randomised to standard therapy or standard therapy with the addition of IV streptokinase within 12 hours of onset of MI. Hospital mortality at 21 days were 10.7% in streptokinase versus 13% in controls with an 18% reduction (p = 0.0002).

GISSI — 1, Lancet 1986

5.3 Beta-Blockers

There are four main effects of beta-blockers on the heart:

- anti-anginal properties
- lowering blood pressure
- treatment of arrhythmias
- to reduce symptoms and enhance survival in heart failure

They work by blocking two types of beta adrenoceptors, B1 and B2.

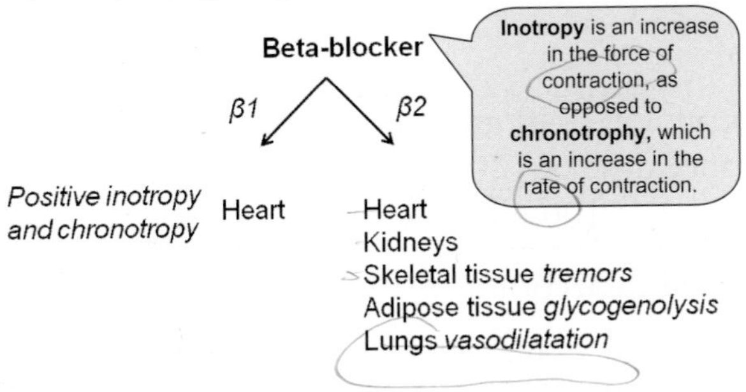

Beta-blocker
Inotropy is an increase in the force of contraction, as opposed to **chronotrophy,** which is an increase in the rate of contraction.
β1
β2
Positive inotropy and chronotropy
Heart
Heart
Kidneys
Skeletal tissue *tremors*
Adipose tissue *glycogenolysis*
Lungs *vasodilatation*

Figure 5.7 The two main types of beta-blockers

The anti-hypertensive effect is brought about by the reduction of cardiac output, reduction of renin from the kidneys and a reduction of sympathetic outflow from the Central Nervous System (CNS) system.

Three main beneficial effects on the heart:

- ↓↓ heart rate — ↑ diastolic perfusion
- ↓ afterload — ↓ wall stress
- ↓ contractility — ↓ O2 demand

Sotalol is a 'special' beta-blocker which has additional effects that make it a Class III anti-arrhythmic. Because of this (and therefore its potential pro-arrhythmic effects) it is not used as a 'standard' beta-blocker for hypertension or angina.

Prescribing beta-blockers

These can be divided into two groups: non-selective and selective beta-blockers. An example of a non-selective beta-blocker is propanolol. Selective beta-blockers include atenolol and metoprolol. There is generally no evidence for any individual superiority within the groups although acceptability may vary according to the different types.

To Impress!

Selective *versus* ***Specific.***

Don't confuse these similar words describing drug-receptor interaction. **Selective** means the drug has a relatively stronger effect on one receptor class than another. **Specific** is a mythical ideal of having an effect purely on one receptor class.

Indications

Cardiovascular uses

- **Angina:**
  - propanolol — 40 mg two to three times daily initially, maintenance dose of 120–240 mg
  - atenolol — 100 mg daily
- **Myocardial infarction:**
  - atenolol — 5 mg intravenous (iv) over 5 minutes within 12 hours of MI, 50 mg orally after 15 minutes, 50 mg after 12 hours then 100 mg daily

- propanolol — prophylaxis after MI, 40mg QDS for 2 days, then 80 mg twice daily
- metoprolol — 5 mg iv every 2 minutes, within 12 hours of MI 50 mg PO after 15 minutes, then QDS for two days. Maintenance dose 200 mg daily in divided doses.

- **Heart failure:**
  - carvedilol — start with 3.125 mg and titrate according
  - bisoprolol — adjunct in stable moderate to severe heart failure, starting regimen:
    - start with 1.25 mg OD and gradually titrate to a maximum dose of 10 mg, over many weeks.

- **Hypertension:**
  - propanolol — 80 mg BD initially, maintenance dose of 60–320 mg daily
  - atenolol — 25–50 mg daily

- **Arrhythmias:** propanolol, bisoprolol, esmolol and sotalol.

Extra-cardiovascular uses

- treatment of glaucoma: timolol eye drops
- symptomatic relief in hyperthyroidism
- prophylaxis in migraine

Contra-indications

- asthma/bronchospasm, although many patients with chronic obstructive pulmonary disease (COPD) can tolerate beta-blockers as long as a cardioselective agent is used
- severe bradycardia high degree heart block
- *severe* claudication
- hypotension
- gangrene or skin necrosis

Side effects

- bronchospasm
- impotence and Raynaud's phenomenon
- exacerbation of renal failure with hydrophilic b-blockers, that is, atenolol, sotalol
- although beta-blockers are not contra-indicated in diabetes, there is some evidence that beta-blockers may mildly worsen glycaemic control and that they mask hypo-glycaemic episodes

CNS effects: worse with *lipid soluble* b-blockers

- fatigue
- nightmares
- depression

Beware of

- Bradycardia
- Hypotension
- Heart failure

Evidence for their use

Beta-blockers improve survivability and reduce symptoms post-MI.

Secondary prevention of Myocardial Infarction

ISIS I (First International Study of Infarct Survival)

Randomised trial comparing atenolol (5–10mg IV immediately followed by 100mg/day PO for 7 days) and placebo amongst 16,027 cases of suspected acute myocardial infarction: For every 200 patients, there was one less death, reinfarction, and cardiac arrest.

Atenolol reduced mortality from MI in the first week by 15%.

ISIS-1. Lancet 1986;2(8498):57–66.

Beta-blockers in Heart failure

CIBIS II (Cardiac Insufficiency Bisoprolol Study II)

A randomised double blinded trial of 2647 patients with heart failure New York Heart Association (NYHA) class III/IV randomly assigned placebo or bisoprolol 1.25 mg daily increasing stepwise to a dose of 10mg. Follow-up period was on average 1.3 years.

Figure 5.8 Secondary prevention of myocardial infarction

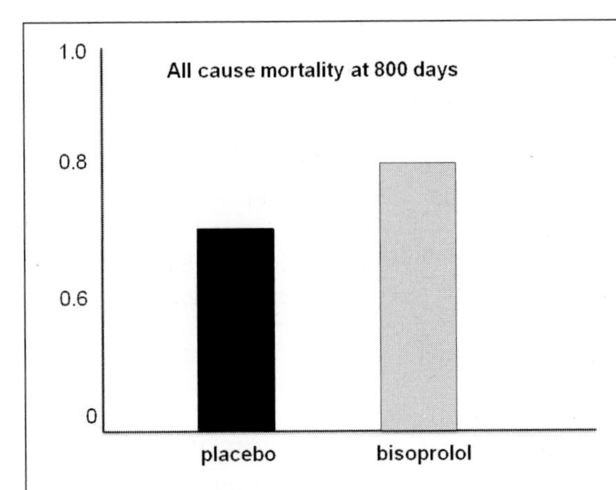

Reduction in:

Death 30%
All cause mortality
All cause hospitalisation due to worsening heart failure.

CIBIS-II Lancet 1999;353: 9–13

Figure 5.9 Comparing mortality between bisoprolol and placebo — The Cardiac Insufficiency Bisoprolol II (CIBIS-II) trial

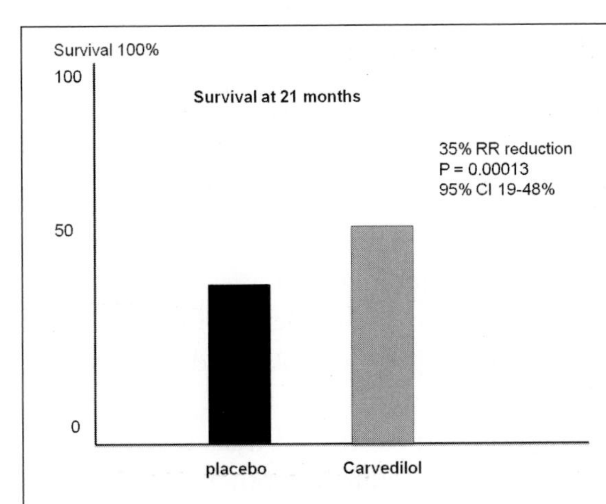

RCT of 2289 patients with heart failure and ejection systolic fraction of <25% on diuretics + ACEi/ARB.

Patients given a placebo or carvedilol showed a significant reduction in all cause mortality in the carvedilol group.

Packer et al., N Engl J Med 2001;344:1651–58

Figure 5.10 Comparing survival between carvedilol and placebo. CORPERNICUS — Carvedilol Prospective Randomised Cumulative Survival trial

UK NICE recommendations

Beta-blockers should be prescribed for left ventricular (LV) systolic dysfunction after ACE inhibitors and diuretic therapy has been initiated.

Start low and go slow with beta-blockers with monitoring of heart rate, blood pressure and clinical status after each titration.

Adverse drug interactions

Beta-blockers are negatively inotropic, and therefore it is generally inadvisable, except in expert hands, to administer them in combination with other negatively inotropic drugs, in particular Diltiazem, Verapamil and Class I anti-arrhythmics such as Propafenone.

Selectivity of beta-blockers in the control of hypertensive patients?

ASCOT-BPLA (the Anglo-Scandinavian cardiac outcomes trial — blood pressure lowering arm)

A randomised controlled trial of 19,257 patients comparing amlodipine and perindopril with atenolol and bendroflumethiazide showed similar reduction endpoints between non-fatal MI and CV death. Note: Although not a statistically significant result, the study also shows that the amlodipine based regimen may be superior to that of the atenolol and bendroflumethiazide regimen.

The ASCOT-BPLA trial showed that the amlodipine-based regimen yielded fewer patients having a non-fatal and fatal stroke, fewer patients having cardiovascular events and fewer patients with diabetes. Two multicentre randomised controlled trials give evidence to suggest that atenolol may be less useful than other beta-blockers in reducing cardiovascular events in hypertensive patients. (*Lancet* 2004;364:1684–9; *Lancet* 2005;366:1545–53)

Beta-blockers and cardiac remodelling (CAPRICORN study)

A study of 1,959 patients with recent MI, all cause mortality was reduced 23%, 15% placebo to 12% carvedilol group. (*Lancet* 2001;357: 1385–90)

Twenty-six patients with dilated cardiomyopathy were randomly assigned metoprolol or standard therapy demonstrated that despite an initial deterioration of systolic function, patients on metoprolol showed a reversal of maladaptive remodelling with a reduction in left ventricular volumes, regression of left ventricular mass and improved ventricular geometry by 18 months. (Hall SA, Cigarroa CG, Marcoux L, *et al.*) Another Australian–New Zealand Randomised Controlled Trial (RCT) study on 415 patients with heart failure due to ischaemic heart disease showed that carvedilol had a beneficial effect on cardiac remodelling; improving left ventricular volumes, left ventricular ejection fraction, and preventing dilatation (Dougherty *et al.* 1997).

5.4 Calcium Channel Blockers (CCB)

Calcium channel blockers affect many cells in the body including cardiac cells, the smooth muscle cells of vessels as well as neuron cells. Their main use in cardiovascular disease is in the treatment of **hypertension** and **supraventricular tachyarrhythmia**. Normally, when an action potential arrives at the myocyte membrane it activates the L-type calcium channel and leads to an overall increase of calcium in the cell. The free calcium binds to the myofilaments resulting in contraction of the cell.

Calcium channel blockers work by inhibiting the L-type calcium channels in the heart leading to a reduction in calcium influx and so decrease the force of contraction. All CCB are vasodilators but not all have an effect on the heart at clinical doses.

They can be divided into:

- **Non-dihydropyridines** have practical actions on the heart (as well as the periphery), and there are only two:
  - *verapamil* — Securon Slow-Release®
  - *diltiazem*: — Tildiem®, Adizem®

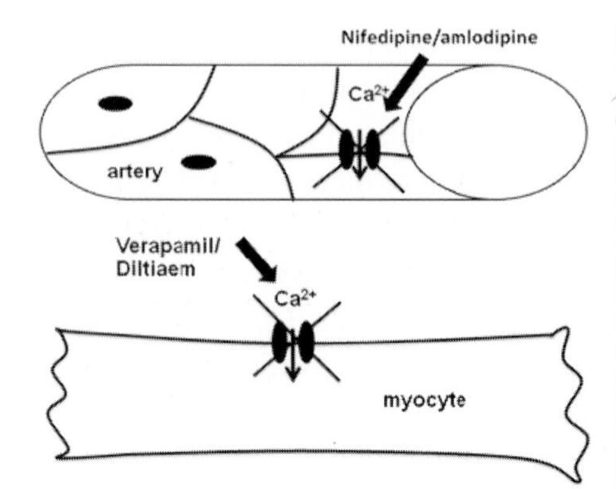

Main effects:

All calcium channel blockers

- vasodilate (peripheral and coronary)

Diltiazem and verapamil additionally have these effects

- negative inotropic effect
- depression of sinus node
- depression of AV node

Figure 5.11 Calcium channel influx

- **Dihydropyridines** which only act on the periphery, and which are numerous, for example:
  - amlodipine — Istin®
  - nifedipine — Adalat®
  - lacidipine

Be careful which type of CCB you use in which condition!

Indications

- angina (particularly when patients are intolerant of ß-blockers)
- hypertension
- supraventricular arrhythmias (*verapamil*)

Contra-indications

All CCB are contra-indicated in,

- hypotension
- heart failure with poor systolic function
- severe aortic stenosis and mitral stenosis

Its vasodilatation effect can cause severe hypotension in these patients!

Verapamil and diltiazem are also contra-indicated in sick sinus syndrome and atrio-ventricular (AV) block.

Side effects

Common:		**Rarer effects:**
Seen in 1–10% of patients due to vasodilatation	• ankle oedema • headaches flushing • constipation • dizziness	• nausea/reflux • myocardial depression • AV block

How do I prescribe calcium channel blockers?

In the treatment of hypertension, you want to ensure that a patient has 24-hour cover. The obvious disadvantage of the immediate-release preparations is that they need to be taken at equally spaced intervals several times throughout the day. Modified released preparations have the advantage that they are released slowly and only need to be given once/twice a day. The disadvantage is that they take time to reach a steady state.

Therefore, when starting an inpatient on verapamil or diltiazem CCB, you can start with the immediate-release preparation and titrate up to an optimal dose for the patient. If administering these drugs intravenously, make sure you have a cardiac monitor with a close eye on blood pressure and heart rate.

Once that is obtained, the patient can be switched to a modified release formula for maintenance. The brands of verapamil and diltiazem vary in their bioavailability (the amount of the drug that gets into the bloodstream, rather than just passing through the gut). Because of this, long-acting verapamil and diltiazem are an exception to the rule of prescribing and documenting medications by generic names: in these two cases, you should name them by brand.

Doses:

Amlodipine

- initially 5 mg OD, increase to 10 mg OD.

Nifedipine

- a very short-acting agent whose use should now largely be replaced by longer-acting agents such as amlodipine. If using this, remember that modified-release doses vary according to manufacturer: check separately for dosage ranges

Verapamil

Supraventricular arrhythmias

- termination: slow IV over 2 to 3 minutes 5–10 mg
- prophylaxis: 40–120 mg PO total dissolved solids (TDS)

Angina or hypertension

- 80–120 mg TDS; or added up into a single once-daily long-acting dose

Diltiazem

Angina

- 60 mg TDS, increase if necessary to 360 mg daily
- again, consult British National Formulary (BNF) re: modified release doses

Evidence for their use

Table 5.2 In angina

TIBET (The Total Ischaemic Burden European Trial)	**APSIS** (The Angina Prognosis Study in Stockholm)
Comparing the use of atenolol, nifedipine and combination therapy in the treatment of chronic stable angina.	Comparing the use of verapamil with metoprolol in patients with stable angina.
Number of patients = 608; 2 years follow-up	Number of patients = 809; 3.4 years follow-up
Results = No difference in cardiac death, fatal MI or unstable angina in all three groups.	Results = No difference in cardiovascular events between the two groups.
Fox KM et al., Eur Heart J 1996	*Rehnqvist N et al., Eur Heart J 1996*

Table 5.3 In hypertension

ALLHAT (Anti-hypertensive and Lipid lowering to prevent heart attack trial)	**INVEST** (International verapamil SR/Tradolapril Study)
Comparing amlodipine versus others (diuretic, ACEi, alpha-blocker) in hypertensive patients. Number of patients: 33,357; 9,048 in amlodipine arm; 4.9 years follow-up	Comparing verapamil +/− ACEi versus atenolol +/− diuretic in hypertensive patients with coronary artery disease. Number of patients: 22,576; 2.7 Years follow-up
Results = No difference in fatal coronary heart disease (CHD) or non-fatal MI between all groups.	Results = Both groups equally effective in reduction of mortality, MI and strokes.
ALLHAT, JAMA 2002;288:2981–97	*Pepine CJ et al., J Am Coll Cardiol 1998;32:1228–37*

Adverse drug reactions

Calcium channel blockers can:

- increase digoxin levels
- increase cyclosporine levels)
- cause asystole when coadministered with beta-blockers especially verapamil.

Advice patients not to drink grapefruit juice as it can affect the metabolism (except amlodipine).

UK NICE Recommendations 2003

Amlodipine should be considered for the treatment of co-morbid hypertension and/or angina in patients with heart failure, but verapamil, diltiazem or short-acting dihydropyridine agents should be avoided.

5.5 Statins

Statins are a hot topic in cardiology and you are likely to be asked questions about their use. They work by inhibiting hydroxymethyl glutaryl (HMG) CoA reductase, the enzyme that catalyses the rate-limiting step responsible for the synthesis of cholesterol in the liver.

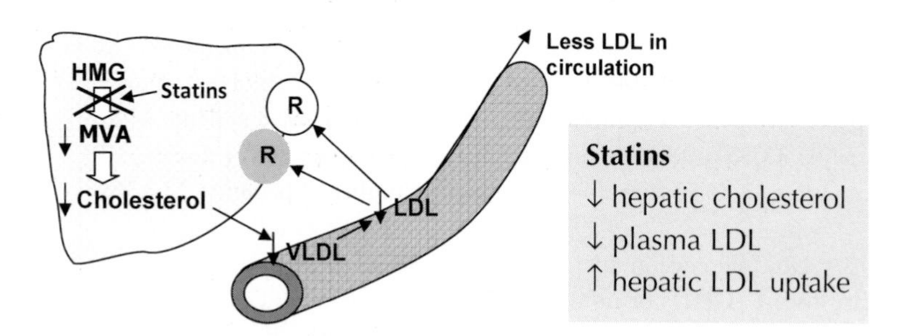

Figure 5.12 Cholesterol metabolism

Figure 5.12 illustrates how statins lower low density lipoprotein (LDL) ('bad' particle that transports cholesterol to tissues) in the blood and it does this more effectively than any other cholesterol-lowering drug. They are, however, less effective at increasing high density lipoprotein (HDL) ('good' particle that transports cholesterol back to liver).

Statins are taken at night because that is when most cholesterol is produced. It is 30% less effective if taken in the morning!

Prescribing information

Simvastatin is the most commonly prescribed statin. The starting dose is usually 10–20 mg orally. The indications for each statin vary slightly but most cardiologists believe in their overall class effect.

Table 5.4 Statins in order of potency

Drug	Trade name	Potency
Rosuvastatin	*Crestor®*	Most
Atorvastatin	*Lipitor®*	
Simvastatin	*Zocor®*	
Pravastatin	*Pravachol®*	Least

Indications

The normal range for blood cholesterol is usually quoted as being between 3.5 and 6.5 mmol/l (the lab reference values vary from hospital to hospital). However, this 'normal' range is a result of Western lifestyle and diet and the cholesterol level should ideally be a lot lower. Each country has their own national targets, and in the UK, the aim is to keep levels <5 mmol/l. This is a set value based on a host of factors including the cost to the NHS of treatment of patients with high cholesterol levels.

Although hypercholesterolaemia is a significant risk factor for cardiovascular disease (CVD), it should not be considered in isolation. Cardiovascular risk should be assessed in combination with age, sex, smoking, BP, diabetes, and family history. This overall percentage risk can be calculated using the Coronary risk prediction charts that can be found at the back of the British National Formulary (BNF) (see also the section *Implications In Primary Care* in Chapter 1 *Clerking Patients*).

> The **UK NICE guidelines** (2006) recommend statins for all patients with a history of CVD and those with a 20% or greater risk of developing coronary heart disease (CHD) in the next 10 years. It is recommended these high-risk patients maintain their cholesterol levels below 4 mmol/l.

Contra-indications

Active liver disease, pregnancy and breast-feeding.

Side effects

> Myoglobin released from damaged muscle cells can be detected as haemoglobin on urine dipstick.

Most of these are dose related. It is quite common for students to blurt out **rhabdomyolysis** when asked about the side effects of statins, but it is important to bear in mind that it is very rare (<0.1%). However, rhabdomyolysis sits on a spectrum of muscle disorders represented below. Symptoms of muscle pain are therefore treated seriously as they can be a precursor to more serious disease.

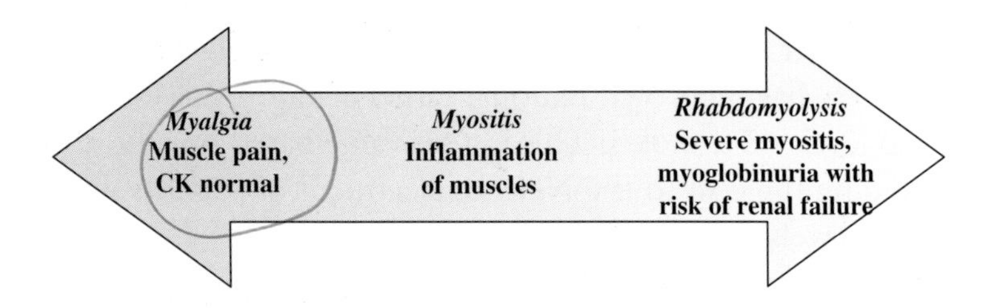

The other serious side effect is **hepatotoxicity** and liver function tests should be checked before initiating therapy. Commoner side effects include headache and gastrointestinal effects such as nausea, vomiting and diarrhoea. Lowering the dose or switching to a different statin can usually resolve these symptoms.

Evidence for their use

There have been many studies on statins, and they have all shown the following benefits:

Figure 5.12 illustrates the vast amount of evidence demonstrating that statins are highly effective at reducing the number of coronary heart events.

- reduction in cardiovascular mortality
- reduction in fatal myocardial infarction (MI) mortality
- reduction in non-fatal stroke
- reduction in unstable angina
- reduction in risk of requiring coronary artery bypass graft (CABG) or primary coronary intervention (PCI)

Prevention of coronary and stroke events in hypertensive patients who do not even have hypercholesterolaemia.

The very first statin mega trial! Four thousand four hundred and forty four patients with moderate hypercholesterolaemia.

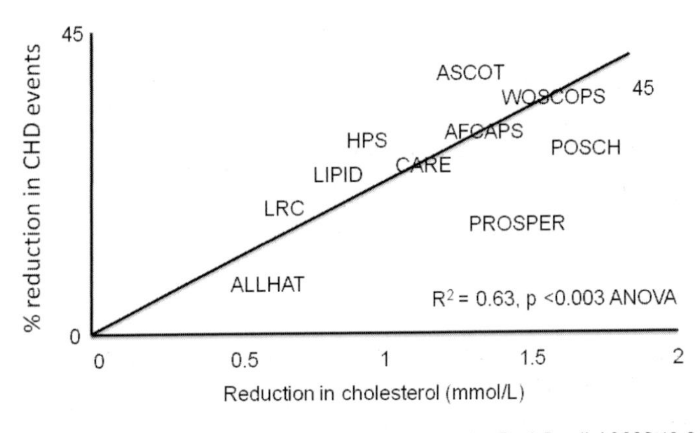

Figure 5.13 Effects of lipid-lowering therapy on coronary heart disease (CHD)

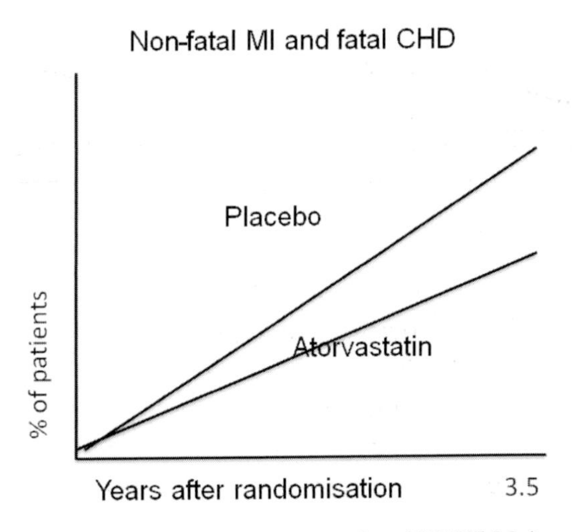

Figure 5.14 Primary prevention ASCOT LLA

Lancet 2003;361:1149–58

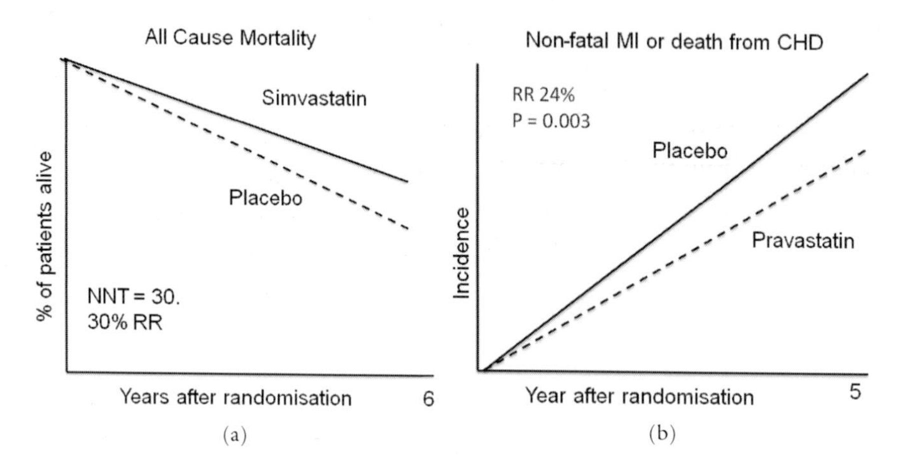

Figure 5.15 (a) Secondary prevention **Scandinavian Simvastatin Survival Study (4S)**; (b) Cholesterol and Recurrent Events Trial (CARE)

Lancet 1994;91:344(8934):1383–9; N Engl J Med 1996;335:1001–9

Four thousand one hundred and fifty nine patients with previous MI and average levels of total and LDL cholesterol.

Note that there is good evidence for the use of statins in both *primary* and *secondary* prevention. All the trials summarised above are multinational, multi-centred randomised control trials.

Adverse drug reactions

Cytochrome P450 inhibitors

- Antibiotics
  - Macrolides, for example, erythromycin
  - Quinolones, for example, ciprofloxacin
- Azole antifungals
- Cyclosporine
- Calcium channel blockers
- Isoniazid
- Cimetidine
- Grapefruit juice

It can be a struggle to remember all the various interactions of different drugs. For statins, the most important ones are related to their route of metabolism. Most statins are prodrugs and are broken down in the liver by the infamous cytochrome P450. Therefore, all P450 inhibitors can potentially induce statin-induced hepatotoxicity and/or rhabdomyolysis. On the other hand, patients taking both statins and warfarin need to be monitored carefully as warfarin levels are increased.

Other means of improving cholesterol levels

It is important to remember that patients on statins should be encouraged to modify their lifestyles as well: the four main being to stop smoking, lose weight, exercise, and enjoy a healthy diet. These are relevant for all aspects of cardiovascular disease!

Lifestyle Modifications
Plant sterols
Fish oils
Nicotinic Acid
Fibrates
Ezetimibe

Ezetimibe is a cholesterol absorption inhibitor that works in the small gut and is used for patients with resistant hypercholesterolaemia. It is usually prescribed in combination with a statin.

Discussion

- Statins given to patients post-myocardial infarction (MI) have been shown to have early beneficial effects suggesting that they have other properties, for example, anti-inflammatory roles in addition to their lipid lowering capacity.
- In countries such as the United States, statins are available over the counter at therapeutic doses. In 2004, simvastatin was made available to the UK public at 10 mg/day. This is controversial in medical circles as there is no evidence to suggest that this low dose is beneficial.
- It is well known that patients with rheumatoid arthritis have a higher risk of cardiovascular complications than the general population. This is believed to be attributable to earlier vessel damage due to the high levels of inflammation in these patients. A 5-year trial starting in 2006 examine whether statins can reduce the excess risk of cardiovascular complications in patients with rheumatoid arthritis, due to their effects of reducing both cholesterol and inflammation.

5.6 Diuretics

Diuretics are often referred to by patients as their 'water tablet'. Diuretics work by increasing urine volume. There are relevant in many fields of medicine but the following chapter will concentrate mainly on their cardiovascular applications. The three types most commonly used in cardiology are:

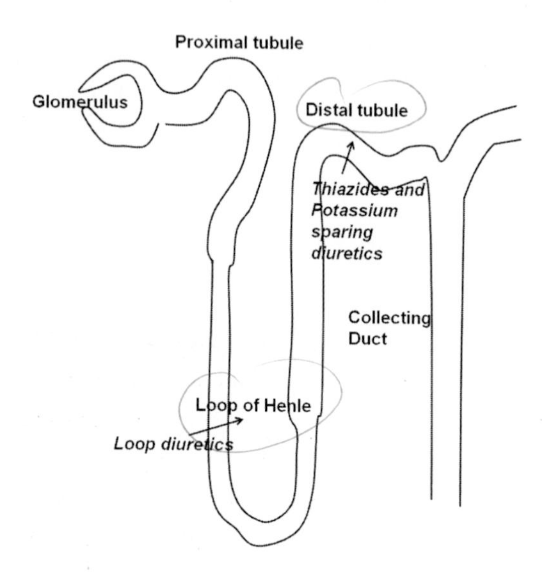

Figure 5.16 Diagram showing where each group of diuretics act on the renal tubules

5.6.1 *Thiazides*

These act on the distal tubular ATPase pumps inhibiting sodium chloride resorption. Water leaves the tubules as it is drawn to the high concentration of solutes in the urine. These drugs can therefore cause hyponatraemia, hypokalaemia, hypercalcaemia and hyperuricaemia. They can also exacerbate diabetes and gout.

> Hypercalcaemia is caused by increased tubular resorption of calcium.

They act within 1–2 hours of administration and their effects can last between 12 and 24 hours. Patients should be advised to take them early in the day so the diuresis doesn't interfere with their sleep.

Doses (for, bendroflumethiazide)

- oedema: initially 5–10 mg PO in the morning daily or on alternative days, maintenance 5–10 mg one to three times weekly
- hypertension: 2.5 mg in the morning

Measure a patient's U&Es prior to initiating a diuretic!

Indications

- oedema
- hypertension

Side effects

- electrolyte imbalances (↓Na, ↓K, ↑Ca)
- diuresis
- postural hypotension
- impotence (reversible)
- gout
- *hyperglycaemia*

Life-threatening complications:

- **pancreatitis**: uncommon but thought to be caused by the drug-induced hypercalcaemia.
- **ventricular arrhythmias**: in susceptible patients exacerbated by the drug-induced hypokalaemia.

Contra-indications

- hypokalaemia, hyponatraemia, hypercalcaemia
- severe renal and hepatic impairment

5.6.2 *Loop diuretics*

Loop diuretics include frusemide and bumetanide. These act on the ascending loop of Henle by inhibiting the co-transport of sodium, chloride and potassium. Both frusemide and bumetanide act within 1 hour of oral administration and the effect lasts for 6 hours. This means that patients can be given this drug twice a day without interfering with sleep at night.

Brand names include: Froop®, Frusid®, Frusol®, and Lasix®

Lasix_onset of action 6 hours!

Doses

- oedema: 40 mg PO initially, 20–40 mg maintenance daily

Indications

- pulmonary oedema due to left ventricular failure
- chronic heart failure
- hypertension resistant to thiazide therapy

Side effects

- diuresis! Huge problem with patient compliance!
- electrolyte imbalance: ↓Na, ↓K, ↓Mg, ↓Ca
- ototoxicity
- postural hypotension
- gastrointestinal disturbance

To Impress!

Patients can develop resistance to loop diuretics of which the mechanism is still unclear but these patients will need their doses increased over time!

Contra-indications

- precomatose states due to liver cirrhosis, renal failure and anuria

Adverse drug interactions

- hypokalaemia can induce toxicity with digoxin and other anti-arrhythmics
- can exacerbate first dose hypotension with ACE inhibitors

5.6.3 *Potassium sparing diuretics and aldosterone antagonists*

Potassium sparing diuretics and aldosterone antagonists include amiloride and spironolactone. These are aldosterone antagonists which prevent resorption of sodium in the distal convoluted tubules. They cause retention of potassium and are therefore often used in conjunction with a thiazide or loop diuretic.

Brand names include: spironolactone — Spirospare®, Aldactone®; amiloride — amilamont®.

Doses

- Congestive heart failure: 25 mg daily has been shown to reduce symptoms and mortality (randomised aldactone evaluation study [RALES])

Indications

- congestive heart failure where patients are at risk of hypokalaemia
- also used in other fluid retentive states, that is:
  - oedema and ascites in cirrhosis
  - malignant ascites
  - nephrotic syndrome

Contra-indications:

- hyperkalaemia
- pregnancy and breast feeding

Adverse drug interactions

There is a risk of hyperkalaemia if prescribed with:

- ACE inhibitors and angiotensin receptor blockers (ARBs)
- Cyclosporine and tacrolimus
- Trimethoprim
- Non-Steroidal Anti-Inflammatory Drugs NSAIDs (by exacerbating renal function)

Side effects

- GI disturbances
- Impotence
- Gynaecomastia
- Menstrual irregularities
- Lethargy, headache, confusion

Evidence for their use

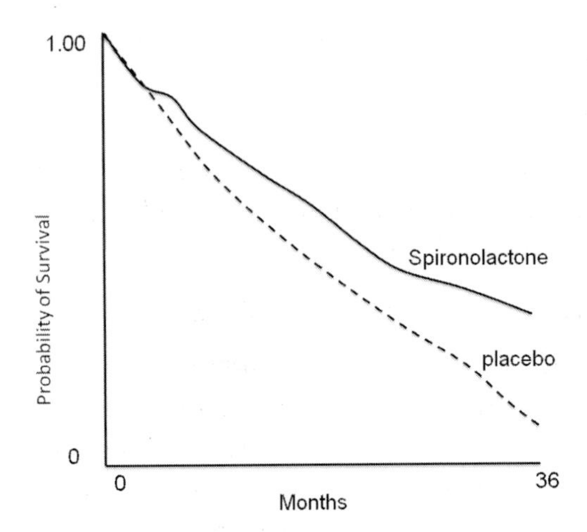

Figure 5.17 RALES (The Randomised Aldactone Evaluation Study Investigators)
Multi-centre, double blinded randomised controlled placebo trial of 1663 patients in NYHA class III/IV severe heart failure with a left ventricular fraction of <35%, and receiving an ACEi, loop diuretic +/− digoxin. Twenty-four-month follow-up. Results showed that spironolactone reduced the risk of death by 30% following a 2-year follow-up.

Pitt et al., N Engl J Med 1999;341:709–17.

5.7 ACE Inhibitors

Angiotensins are potent vasoconstricting agents involved in the renin-angiotensin system (RAS). By constricting blood vessels, they increase resistance to blood flow (total peripheral resistance — TPR) thus increasing the blood pressure. ACE inhibitors work by inhibiting angiotensin converting enzyme (ACE) which converts angiotensin I to angiotensin II. Inhibiting ACE activity reduces total peripheral resistance which widens the blood vessels; thereby ACE inhibitors reduce blood pressure.

Reduction in total peripheral resistance reduces the blood pressure which decreases the myocardial oxygen consumption. This improves cardiac output and moderates left ventricular and vascular hypertrophy.

This is why ACE inhibitors are indicated in the management of heart disease (see below).

Prescribing ACE inhibitors

Commonly prescribed ACE inhibitors you should be familiar with are listed below along with their trade names. **Hint**: For any drug that ends in '*pril*', think ACE inhibitor.

Drug		*Trade Name*
Captopril	—	*Capoten®*
Enalapril	—	*Innovace®*
Lisinopril	—	*Cardace®*, *Zestril®*
Perindopril	—	*Coversyl®*
Ramipril	—	*Tritace®*

Monitoring treatment

Check the patient's **renal function** (that is, urea and electrolytes [U&Es]) before starting treatment and after each significant dose increase. Start the ACE inhibitor at a low dose to avoid hypotension and hyperkalaemia.

Indications

Consultants expect you to know at least the following:

- Hypertension
- Heart failure
- Left ventricular dysfunction
- Acute MI within 24 hours (see ISIS-4 below)
- Diabetic nephropathy (can reduce proteinuria)

Contra-indications

The main ones are:

- Pregnancy (birth defects in second/third trimester)
- Renal artery stenosis
- Hyperkalaemia (↑K^+ due to aldosterone antagonism)
- Hypotension

Side effects

When asked the side effects of any drug, always list the **common ones first**.

- **Dry cough** — seen in up to 20% of patients
- **Hyperkalaemia** — due to antagonism of aldosterone
- **Hypotension** — first dose hypotension is commonest in short-acting agents like Captopril
- Angioedema
- Skin rash
- Taste disturbance

ACE inhibitors also inhibit *Kinase II* — the enzyme that breaks down bradykinins in the lungs. Bradykinins accumulate irritating the airway resulting in a **DRY cough!**

Patients intolerant to ACE-I should try an **Angotensin-II receptor antagonist**, that is, Losartan (see Drug section on ARBs).

Evidence for their use

HOPE and **EUROPA** are common 'dinner table names' amongst cardiologists. Both are trials on **primary prevention*** of CVD. Heart Outcomes Prevention Evaluation (HOPE) is a randomised controlled trial involving more than 4,000 patients (see below for results). In the EUROPA study of patients with stable coronary artery disease (CAD), perindopril 8 mg daily was associated with a significant absolute risk reduction (ARR) of 1.9% in the reduction of death from MI and cardiac arrest compared to placebo.

Use post-myocardial infarction

By reducing the work-load of the heart, ACE inhibitors increase survival rates in patients who have suffered a myocardial infarction.

Alongside aspirin and a beta-blocker, an ACE inhibitor should be started *within the first 24 hours of an MI.* The rationale for their use is evident from both the **ISIS-4** trial (below) and the **GISSI-3** trial. In the GISSI-3 trial, randomising patients on Lisinopril for six weeks post-MI reduced their mortality rates from 19.3% (placebo) to 18.1%.

ACE inhibitors should be used with caution in the following situations.

- **Impaired renal function** — see Renal artery stenosis and the triple whammy effect below.
- **Potassium supplements** — ACE-I also increase potassium levels!
- **Lithium** — by increasing the blood concentration of Lithium, ACE-I increases their side effect.
- **Aortic stenosis** or **cardiac outflow obstruction** — these patients are unable to increase their cardiac output.
- **Hypovolaemia OR Dehydration** — the vasodilatation induced by ACE-I may exacerbate these conditions.

Renal artery stenosis and the triple whammy effect

In bilateral **renal artery stenosis** (or unilateral stenosis if there is only one functional kidney), ACE inhibitors prevent the efferent arterioles in the glomerulus from constricting, which reduces the glomerular filtration rate (GFR) exacerbating the renal impairment. This effect is worse in patients on a Non-Steroidal Anti-Inflammatory Drug (**NSAID**) and a **Diuretic** — the so-called 'triple whammy' effect; such patients are at very high risk of developing renal failure.

Primary prevention
HOPE

Ramipril reduced the total number of cardiovascular events (heart attack, stroke, or cardiovascular death) by 22% in patients with predisposing cardiac risk factors (diabetes, ischaemic heart disease, peripheral vascular disease or stroke).

Secondary prevention
ISIS 4

In ISIS-4, mortality rate for oral captopril was compared with oral mononitrate, and iv magnesium in patients with heart attack. Mortality rates at five weeks were significantly better with ACE inhibitors (7.19%) than with placebo (7.69%).

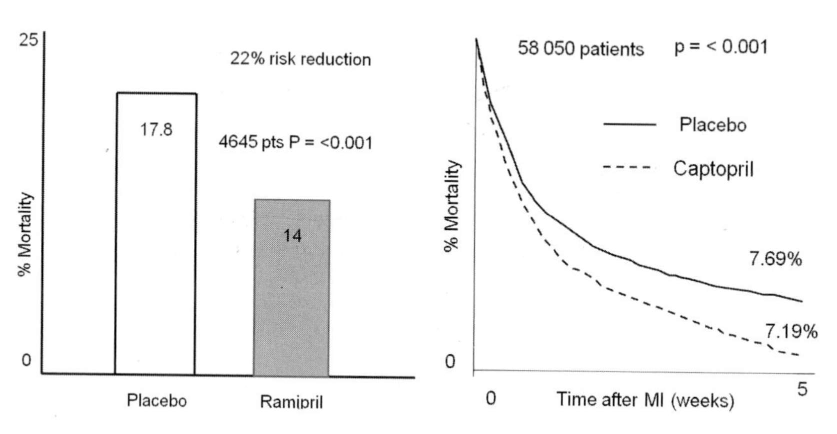

Figure 5.18 Comparing ACE inhibitor with placebo
HOPE. N Engl J Med 2000;342:145–53; ISIS 4. Lancet 1995;18:345(8951):669–85

5.8 Angiotensin II Receptor Antagonists

Angiotensin II receptor antagonists/angiotensin receptor blockers act by blocking AT1 receptors.

Indications

- hypertension
- heart failure with impaired left ventricular function

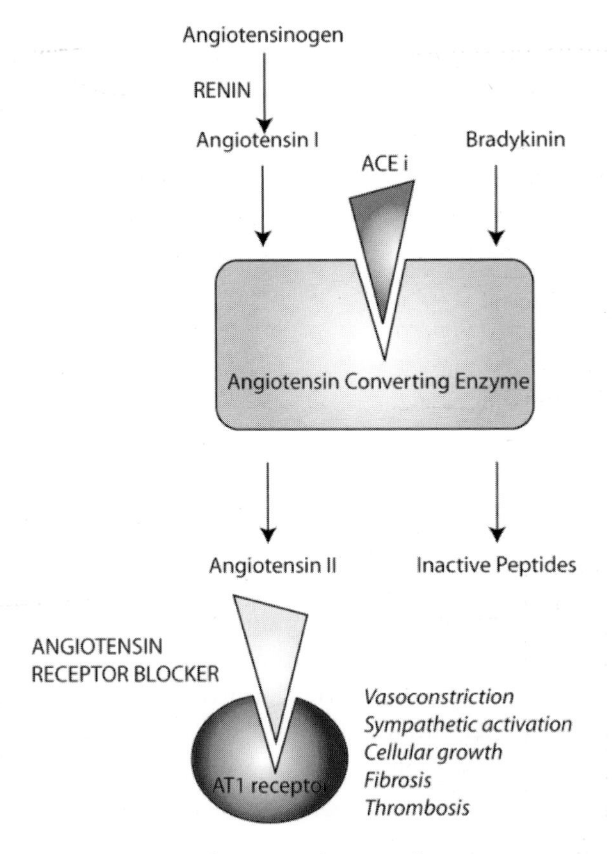

Figure 5.19 Mechanism of action

- alternative to ACE inhibitors (in patients who have ACEI induced cough)

Examples

- candesartan — *Amias*®, irbesartan — *Aprovel*®, + diuretic — *Co-Aprovel*®, losartan — *Cozaar*®, valsartan — *Diovan*

Caution in: Renal artery stenosis — monitoring of plasma K^+ is advised.

Table 5.5 Side effects and contra-indications of angiotensin II receptor antagonists

Side effects (usually mild)	Contra-indications
• symptomatic hypotension, for example, dizziness • hyperkalaemia • angioedema	• pregnancy • severe aortic/mitral stenosis

Evidence for its use

Secondary prevention

ELITE (Evaluation of Losartan In The Elderly study)
Randomisation of 722 patients to losartan 50 mg OD and captopril 50 mg TDS in patients with symptomatic heart failure and left ventricular dysfunction. Early study showed losartan was superior to captopril in terms of mortality and morbidity but later study showed no difference between the two. [hazard ratio losartan: captopril 1.13, 95% confidence interval (CI) 0.95/–1.35, $P = 0.16$]

Composite of mortality and hospitalization from all causes were 752 and 707 events respectively (hazard ratio 1.07, 95% CI 0.96–1.18, $P = 0.21$).

Lancet 1997;349:747–52

Adverse drug interactions

ARBs will potentiate other anti-hypertensives. Be careful of the risk of hypotension when ARBs are teamed with diuretics. They can also exacerbate hyperkalaemia when used in combination with a potassium sparing drug and may cause renal failure when used with an NSAID.

5.9 Anti-arrhythmics

Anti-arrhythmic drugs can be classified according to where they act on the heart. They can also be classified according to their effects on the electrical behaviour of the myocardial cells. Remember all anti-arrhythmic drugs can cause arrhythmias!

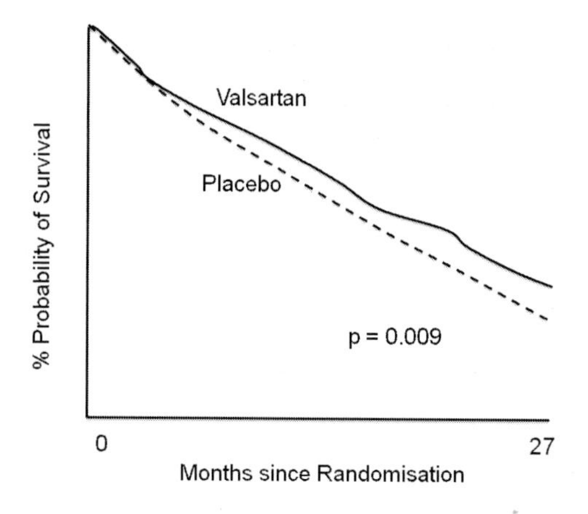

Five thousand and ten patients with New York Heart Association (NYHA) class II, III, or IV were randomly assigned to receive 160 mg of valsartan or placebo twice daily. The primary outcomes were mortality and the combined end point of mortality and morbidity, defined as the incidence of cardiac arrest with resuscitation, hospitalisation for heart failure, or receipt of intravenous inotropic or vasodilator therapy for at least 4 hours. Overall mortality was similar in the two groups.

Figure 5.20 VeHT (Valsartan Heart Failure Trial)

Cohn JN et al., New Engl J Med 2001;345:1667–75

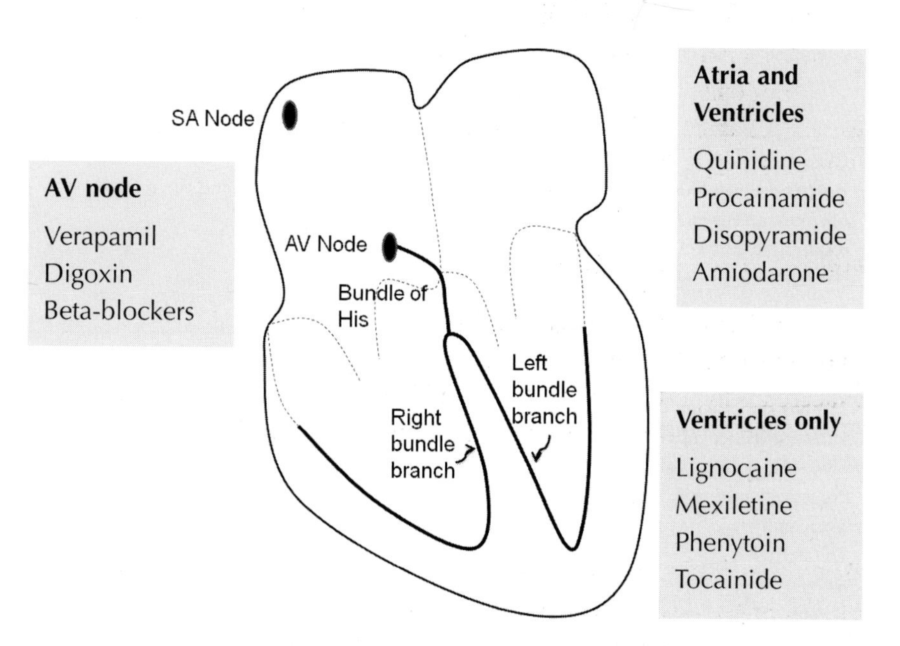

Figure 5.21 Where the drugs act

Vaughn-Williams Classification

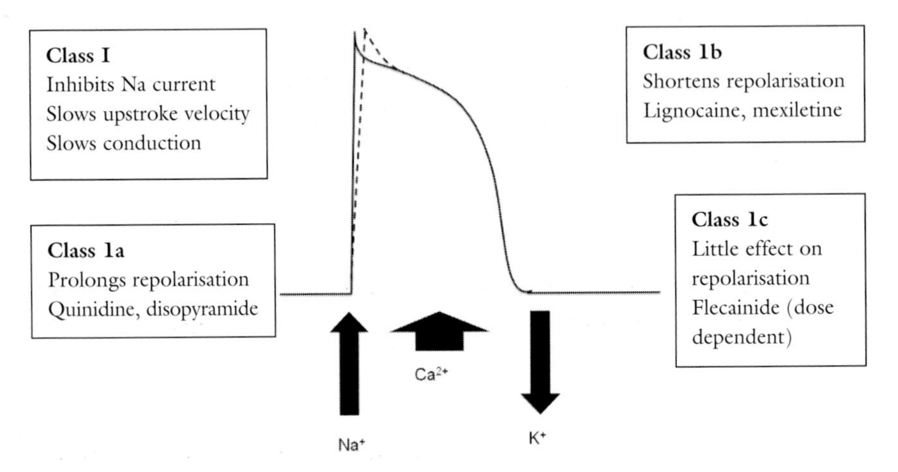

Figure 5.22 Action potential

The steep upstroke of the AP is due to the fast influx of Na into the cell. The plateau phase is due to the influx of Ca via slow Ca channels and the efflux of potassium. During the down sloping stage, Ca channels close while K channels stay open.

Class II
B-adrenoceptor blockade inhibits calcium current in AV node cells resulting in slows AV node conduction

Class III
Prolong repolarisation and the refractory period
Amiodarone
Sotalol
Bretylium

Class IV
Inhibits the calcium current in cardiac muscle
Effects cells dependent on Ca current
Slows AV node conduction
Negatively inotropic
Verapamil
Diltiazem

5.9.1 *Supraventricular tachycardias*

Adenosine

This can be used to slow down a supraventricular tachycardia so that the underlying rhythm can be identified. It has a half-life of 8–10 seconds.

Dose

- rapid bolus of 6 mg intravenously into a central or large peripheral vein followed by another 6mg after 1–2 minutes if necessary.

Side effects

It is important to warn patients that they may experience nausea, chest discomfort and flushing sometimes referred to as 'feelings of impending doom!' Adenosine can cause bronchospasm in patients with asthma.

Contra-indications

- second or third degree AV block
- sick sinus syndrome
- Caution if patients are on carbamazepine, theophyllines and dipyridamole.

5.9.2 *Supraventricular and ventricular arrhythmias*

Amiodarone

This drug is often considered the miracle anti-arrhythmic drug. It can be used when other drugs are ineffective or contra-indicated and is useful in paroxysmal supraventricular, nodal, ventricular tachycardias, atrial fibrillation, flutter and ventricular fibrillation.

This drug has a very *long half-life* and only needs to be given once daily. It requires a loading dose and takes many weeks or months to achieve a steady plasma concentration.

Side effects

Remember the *6Ps:*

Prolongs action potential duration
Photosensitivity and microdeposits in the cornea
Pigmentation of skin
Peripheral neuropathy
Pulmonary alveolitis and fibrosis
Peripheral conversion of T4 to T3 is inhibited –> hypothyroidism

> Prior to prescribing amiodarone, patients must have their eyes checked thyroid and liver functions checked and rechecked at 6 months. A chest X-ray should also be obtained prior to initiating treatment.

This drug has many adverse drug interactions, therefore always check in the British National Formulary (BNF) if you're unsure.

5.9.3 *Ventricular arrhythmias*

Lidocaine (lignocaine)

This is administered by slow IV injection for the termination of ventricular arrhythmias during emergencies. It can be given following an MI. It has a short duration of action (15–20 minutes) following IV injection.

Side effects

- dizziness
- paraesthesia
- drowsiness
- respiratory depression
- convulsions
- hypotension and bradycardia

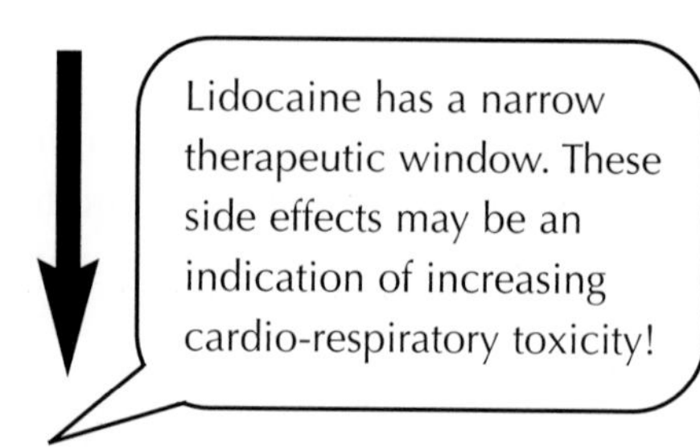

Contra-indications

- sino-atrial disorders
- AV block
- severe myocardial depression
- porphyria

Digoxin

Digoxin is the most commonly used cardiac glycoside and acts by increasing the force of myocardial contraction and reducing conductivity within the AV node by activity on the Na/K pump. It has a *long half-life of 36 hours* and is generally not suitable for acute management of arrhythmias.

Adverse effect of the drug is both dependent on its concentration in plasma as well as the sensitivity of the conducting system or of the myocardium. Special attention must be given when prescribing to elderly patients.

A plasma level of 1–2.6 nmols is desirable and regular monitoring is not considered necessary unless toxicity is suspected. It can cause ECG changes including ST depression and T wave depression. Hypokalaemia predisposes patients to toxicity as digoxin competes with K for the same binding site on the Na/K pump. Be extra careful with patients on diuretics and other drugs that cause hypokalaemia. Measurement of potassium level is important prior to starting digoxin treatment. Digoxin toxicity can be reversed by discontinuing the drug or with digoxin specific antibody fragments (Digibind®).

Brand names

Lanoxin®

Indications

- supraventricular arrhythmias especially persistent AF
- symptomatic use in heart failure (RADIANCE)

Side effects

Remember all anti-arrhythmics are pro-arrhythmics!

Despite xanthopsia being the side effect medical students most commonly remember, don't forget the commoner side effects also!

- anorexia
- nausea and vomiting
- diarrhoea and abdominal pain
- headaches, drowsiness, confusion, dizziness
- visual disturbances, for example, xanthopsia (yellow discoloration)
- gynaecomastia.

Contra-indications

- intermittent complete heart block
- second degree AV block
- supraventricular arrhythmias caused by Wolff-Parkinson-White (WPW) syndrome
- ventricular tachycardia/ventricular fibrillation
- hypertrophic cardiomyopathy

Adverse drug interactions

Digoxin is excreted in the kidneys. Any drug that interferes with this will cause varying degrees of digoxin retention. These include:

- amiodarone
- verapamil
- itraconazole

In 10% of patients, digoxin will be metabolised by a gut bacterium. Drugs that interfere with this breakdown include:

- erythromycin
- clarithromycin
- tetracycline

Evidence for its use

RADIANCE (The Randomised Assessment of Digoxin on Inhibitors of Angiotensin Converting Enzyme trial)

A double-blinded, randomised controlled placebo study of heart failure patients (Class II/III) in which 93 withdrew their use of digoxin whilst 85 continued with its use. There were more patients with worsening heart failure in the withdrawal group ($p = < 0.001$). There was, however, no change in mortality.

Packer et al., N Engl J Med 1993;329:1–7

Table 5.6 Summary table

	AF/A Flutter/SVT	AVNRT	AV node
	Disopyramide Amiodarone	Vagal manoeuvres	β-blockers
Rate control	Digoxin CCB β-blockers	Verapamil β-blockers	Flecainide Amiodarone
Prophylaxis	Amiodarone Disopyramide Procainamide	Digoxin Flecainide	Disopyramide Quinidine Procainamide Sotalol

5.10 Nitrates

Mechanism of action

Organic nitrates act by relaxing smooth muscle and causing vasodilatation. Glyceryl trinitrate (GTN) and other organic nitrates need to be converted into nitric oxide before it can act by increasing Cyclic Guanosine Monophosphate (cGMP). This leads to a decrease in arterial pressure hence cardiac output and myocardial oxygen consumption. They have no effect on the disease process.

Indications

- prophylatic and short term control of angina

> **NB:** GTN has a short shelf life and needs to be replaced every 3 months.

Contra-indications

- aortic stenosis
- hypertrophic obstructive cardiomyopathy
- nitrate resistance (more common in diabetics)

Route

- sublingual
  - GTN, 0.4 mg abate attack within 3–5 minutes
- oral
  - isosorbide mono (30–240 mg) and dinitrate
- transdermal patches

Side effects

- tachycardia
- headaches (due to cerebral arterial vasodilatation)
- tolerance in the long term

5.11 Potassium Channel Openers

Mechanism of action

Activation of potassium channels on the heart causes an efflux of potassium ions resulting in hyperpolarisation of myocyte. This in turn inhibits calcium influx into the cell. The reduction of calcium ions in the cell causes relaxation and vasodilatation.

Indication

- prevention and long-term management of angina

Contra-indications

- not for use in acute angina or acute coronary syndromes
- care with patients taking hypoglycaemics which act via potassium channels

Prescribing information

- initially 10 mg BD, maintenance 10–20 mg BD

Side effects

- headaches
- flushing
- hypotension
- tachycardia

UK NICE Recommendations 2003

Amlodipine should be considered for the treatment of co-morbid hypertension and/or angina in patients with heart failure, but verapamil, diltiazem or short-acting dihydropyridine agents should be avoided.

Adverse drug interactions

Do not use in combination with Sildenafil (Viagra) as this will cause severe hypotension.

Chapter 6

In Theatre

This section aims to equip you with a broad understanding of cardiac anatomy, taking you through the layers of the myocardium through to its blood and nervous supply. In addition, the section on coronary artery bypass grafting (CABG) gives an overall understanding of what is involved in the operation.

6.1 Anatomy of the Heart

The heart is a fist sized muscular pump which sits behind the sternum between the second to sixth costal cartilages at the level of T5–8. Figure 6.1 shows the gross anatomy of the heart and the main coronary vessels.

As you can see from Fig. 6.1, the left border of the heart comprises of the left ventricle. The inferior border of the heart is mainly comprised of the right ventricle and the right border of the heart is mainly the right atrium.

The heart is supplied by the right and left coronary arteries that arise from the ascending aorta just beyond where the aortic valve sits.

Layers of the heart (from superficial to deep)

- epicardium
- myocardium
- endocardium

Pericardium

- fibrous pericardium (outermost)
- serous pericardium
    - parietal layer
    - visceral layer (= epicardium)

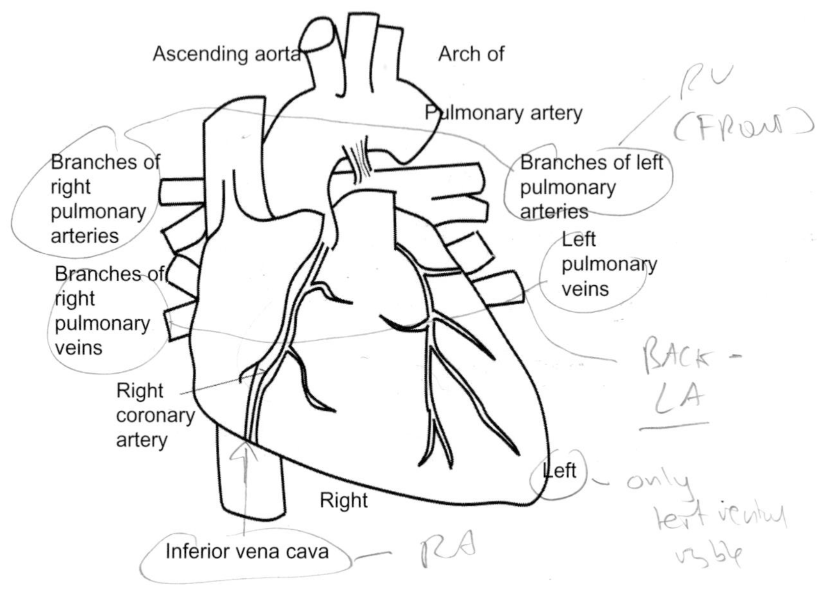

Figure 6.1 Anatomy of the heart

The left coronary artery divides into the left anterior descending artery and the circumflex artery. The left anterior descending artery supplies the interventricular septum and anterior walls of both ventricles. The coronary artery supplies the left atrium and posterior wall of the left ventricle.

The right coronary artery sits in the coronary sinus (atrioventricular groove) around the right margin of the heart and becomes the posterior interventricular artery which supplies the posterior wall of both ventricles.

In the majority of people, the right coronary artery is dominant. However, the left coronary artery is dominant in 15% of people.

The heart is innervated by the sympathetic and parasympathetic nervous system. The right and left vagus nerves innervate the sinoatrial node (SA) and atrioventricular node (AV) respectively.

There are four heart valves: the mitral and aortic valves on the left and tricuspid and pulmonary on the right. The pulmonary and aortic valves are semilunar valves due to their 'moonlike' cusps. The mitral valve only has two cusps and is called a biscupid valve.

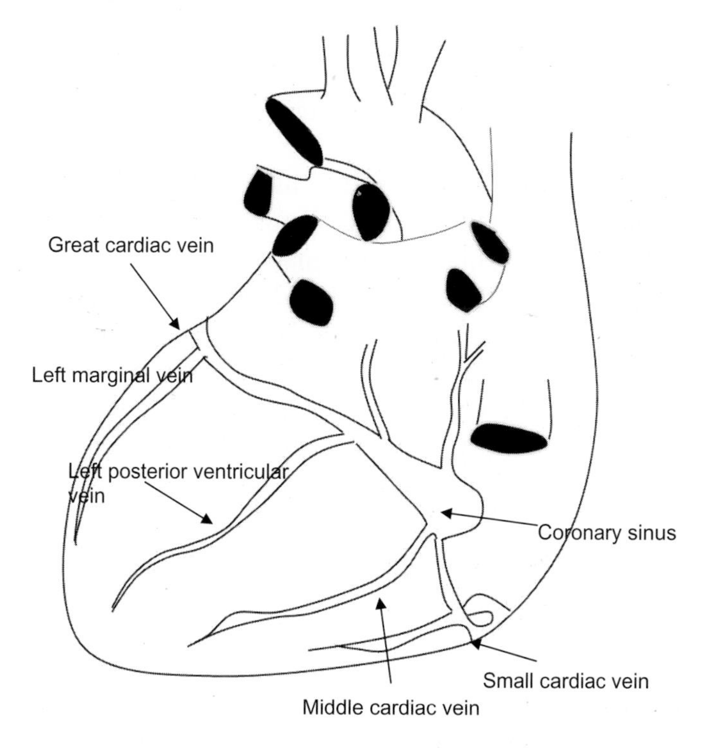

Figure 6.2 Veins of the heart

Blood from the anterior surface of the heart drains into the great cardiac vein whilst blood from the posterior surface drains into the middle cardiac vein. Collectively, they drain into the coronary sulcus and empty into the right atrium.

6.2 Patients Having Coronary Artery Bypass Graft (CABG)

Patients suitable for this operation may fall into one of the following categories:

- **chronic stable angina** inadequately controlled by medical therapy
- **unstable angina**

- **coronary artery disease in association with other cardiac disease**, for example, valvular disease
- **following complications of percutaneous coronary intervention**

The EuroSCORE system is widely used in the UK to stratify the risk of the procedure. The main risk factors include chronic obstructive pulmonary disease, obesity and renal dysfunction.

There are many techniques employed for this operation. There is evidence to show that the use of the left internal mammary artery (LIMA) is superior to the use of a saphenous vein graft in terms of a reduction in cardiac events including angina, myocardial infarction (MI) and sudden death. It maintains its arterial and venous connections to the subclavian vessels. It is generally used to replace the left anterior descending and its diagonal branches although other arteries such as the right internal mammary and the radial artery can also be used. Venous grafts also run the risk of atherosclerotic plaques developing within 12 months. The reasons for the thickening of the vessel wall is two-fold: a) the loss of nourishment due to the absence of a vasa vasora leads to hyperplasia of the media and intima and b) the increased stress on the vessel wall once it is in the arterial circulation.

6.2.1 *Complications*

The Coronary Artery Surgery Study in the USA and the European coronary surgery study reported overall survival following CABG to be 95% at 1 year, and 7% at 10 years. In the UK, the mortality associated with this operation has been increasing as CABG is being more and more reserved for complex cases with straightforward cases being handled by percutaneous coronary intervention (PCI). The figure is quoted as 3%. Other complications include:

- Stroke (2%): it is important to check for a carotid bruit and some doctors advocate operating on stenoses of more than 75% prior to the bypass operation

- Chest infections
- Atelectasis
- Wound infections
- Atrial fibrillation (one-third of patients)
- MI (uncommon)

6.2.2 *Preparation prior to theatre*

In addition to bloods, an electrocardiogram (ECG) and an angiogram are the bare minimum, the patient will need to be examined for other risk factors and followed up with the necessary investigations.

The work-up includes:

- ECG
- Chest X-ray (CXR) for both cardiac and lung pathologies and comparison with post-operative films
- Pulmonary function test (PFT) to assess pulmonary reserve
- Urea and electrolytes (U&Es)
- Full blood count (FBC)
- Glucose
- Coagulation screen
- Cross match 4 units of blood
- MRSA swabs
- Angiography

6.2.3 *The operation*

This is a 2–3 hour operation done under general anaesthesia and is divided into two stages. The first stage involves the harvest of the graft. In the second stage, the patient needs to be heparinised and the right atrium and upper ascending aorta needs to be cannulated. During the procedure, a transient state of ischaemia is induced by cross-clamping the ascending aorta and reducing the body temperature to 32 degrees Celsius to minimise myocardial damage.

One of the major recent advances in coronary bypass surgery has been the development of beating heart bypass surgery, also called ‘off-pump’ surgery. Other developments include minimally invasive surgery and robotic surgery which allows for smaller incisions and faster patient recovery.

6.2.4 *Post-operation*

Post-CABG, patients are ventilated for 3–4 hours and extubated when stable. These patients require cardiac rehabilitation follow-up including lifestyle modification of risk factors, and maintaining blood pressure and cholesterol within normal limits.

Chapter 7

Management Cribsheets

Welcome to the quick reference section. The following pages contain management flow sheets for common/emergency cardiac presentations. We have summarised the steps allowing easy access, particularly during those precarious moments when you are faced with the unwell patient. Further details are available in Chapter 4 *Commonly Encountered Patients.*

Always begin management of the acutely unwell patient with ABCs — airway, breathing, circulation. Use the adult life support (ALS) algorithm in Fig. 7.1 in unresponsive patients.

7.1 Management of Acute Pulmonary Oedema

Breathlessness in acute left ventricular failure (LVF), results from accumulation of fluid in the alveolar space causing impaired gaseous exchange.

7.1.1 *Initial management*

The aim is to relieve the initial symptoms of breathlessness.

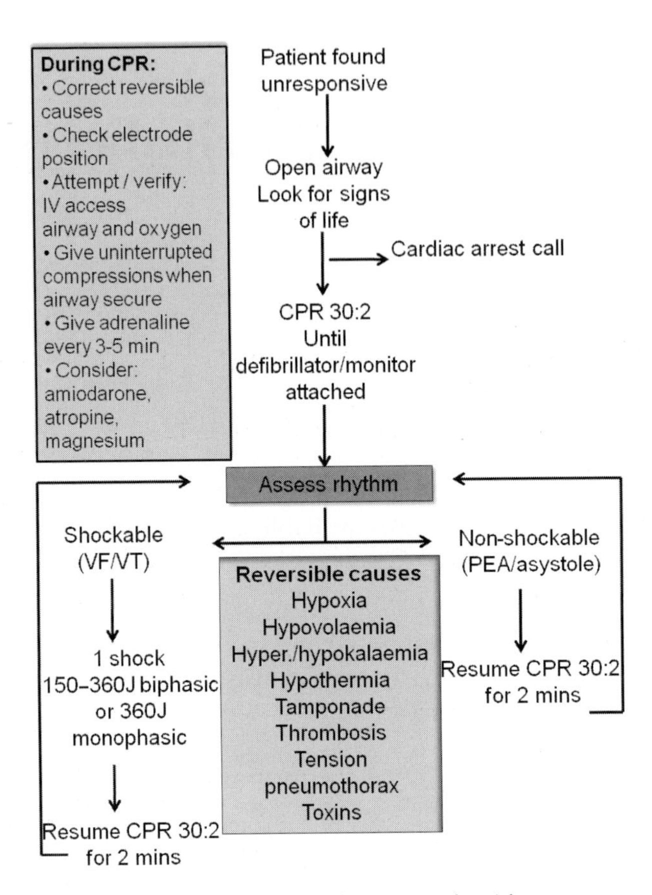

Figure 7.1 Adult life support algorithm

Sit patient up

↓

Give 100% oxygen

↓

Intravenous (IV) access + electrocardiogram (ECG) monitoring +
order chest radiograph X-ray (CXR)
(send bloods including cardiac enzymes and arterial blood gas)

↓

5 mg IV morphine + anti-emetic

↓

40–80 mg IV frusemide

↓

2 puffs glyceryl trinitrate (GTN)

If symptoms persist, consider an infusion of GTN
or frusemide (follow local hospital protocol).
In patients with low cardiac output, inotropes such as
dobutamine/dopamine may be used to increase cardiac
output and contractility.

Main Causes:

- **M**yocardial infarction/Ischaemic Heart Disease
- **C**ardiomyopathies
- **V**alvular disease

Features:

- sudden shortness of breath (SOB) relieved by sitting/standing up
- wheeze
- orthopnoea/paroxysmal nocturnal dyspnoea (PND)
- frothy sputum

Alveolar oedema (Bat's wings)

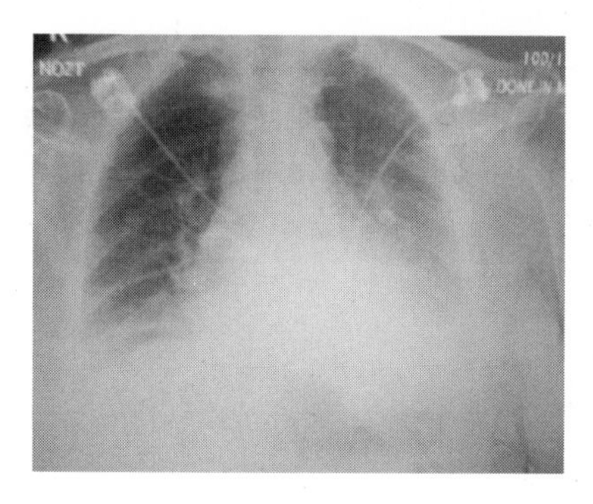

Kerley **B** lines

Dilated upper vessels

Cardiomegaly

Pleural **E**ffusions

Figure 7.2 The ABCs of pulmonary oedema on chest radiograph (see 'commonly encountered patients' — heart failure)

7.1.2 *Principles of management*

- Opiate (morphine/diamorphine) — this helps to relieve the patient's anxiety and may also vasodilate thus reducing the preload and afterload.
- Loop diuretic (frusemide) — initial mode of action is to vasodilate thereby reducing the circulatory volume (preload), action on the ascending limb of the loop of Henle results in diuresis.
- Venodilators (GTN) — these reduce both preload and afterload. Note: Monitor blood pressure (BP); aim to keep systolic BP above 90 mmHg.

7.2 Management of Acute Coronary Syndromes

Acute coronary syndrome is an umbrella term that covers both ST-elevation myocardial infarction (STEMI) and non-ST elevation MI (NSTEMI) including Q wave MI. The diagram below is useful in classifying the different types of acute coronary syndromes. It is important to consider the likely cause.

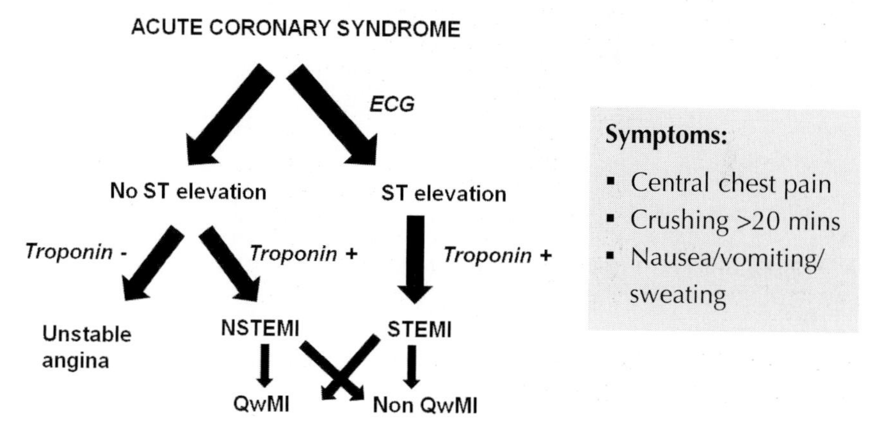

Figure 7.3 Adapted from *Oxford Handbook of Acute Medicine*, 2nd edition

In terms of management, patients can be broadly classified into those with STEMI and those with NSTEMI. Investigations and management should really be conducted simultaneously.

7.2.1 *Management of STEMI*

As with the management of any medical emergency, always start with attention to **A**irway, **B**reathing and **C**irculation.

> Forty per cent die within 24 hours; 2–8% die in hospital; 10% die after the first year.

Airway — 100% oxygen

↓

Breathing + ECG monitoring

↓

Circulation (*insert two large bore cannulas into the antecubital fossae and take bloods including full blood count [FBC], urea and electrolytes [U&Es], troponin, lipids and glucose*)

↓

Give 300 mg aspirin orally

↓

5–10 mg morphine + 10 mg metoclopramide

↓

2 puffs GTN

↓

Beta-blocker if not contra-indicated (that is, in asthma)

↓

ECG demonstrates ST elevation

- **>1 mm in two adjacent limb leads**
- **>2 mm in two adjacent chest leads**
- **New onset left bundle branch block (LBBB)**
- **Posterior infarct with ST depression in V1–3**

↓

Percutaneous coronary intervention (PCI) in primary centre/thrombolysis

7.2.2 *Contra-indications to thrombolysis*

- Previous haemorrhagic stroke
- Stroke or cerebrovascular accident (CVA) within 6 months
- Active internal bleeding
- Aortic dissection
- Recent major surgery or trauma
- Bleeding disorder

7.2.3 *Post-reperfusion therapy*

Following PCI or thrombolysis, the patient will need anti-thrombotic therapy to keep the arteries open usually with a low molecular weight heparin (LMWH) and the addition of aspirin and clopidogrel. If there are no contra-indications, these patients would also benefit from a beta-blocker, ACE inhibitor and statin therapy (see Chapter 5- 'Drugs'). Patients will need daily examination for complications, serial ECGs and cardiac markers over the next couple of days.

7.2.4 *Complications*

DIGAMI (Diabetes Mellitus, Insulin Glucose Infusion in Acute Myocardial Infarction) Study

This study suggests that aggressive blood glucose control (that is, via insulin-glucose infusion/subcutaneous insulin) during and subsequent to a myocardial infarction, has beneficial prognostic implications.

Thus, patients should be commenced on dextrose/insulin infusion post-MI. The leading cause of death in patients with diabetes is myocardial infarction!

Remember:

METFORMIN should be STOPPED following an MI due to the increase risk of lactic acidosis (MI → tissue hypoxia → anaerobic respiration → lactic acid production).

It is important to consider the likely causes in relation to the time since their presentation of symptoms. Therefore, complications should be categorised into those occurring **hours**, **days** or **weeks** following a heart attack.

Table 7.1 Complications post-myocardial infarction

Hours	Hours/Days	Days/Weeks
• Ventricular arrhythmias • Failed reperfusion	• Cardiac rupture • Reinfarction • Ventricular septal defect • Papillary muscle rupture — mitral regurgitation — left ventricular rupture	• Thromboembolism • Chronic heart failure • Ventricular tachycardia • Dressler's syndrome

However, when stumped for an answer on the complications, the mnemonic below may be useful. Remember that the commonest complication is actually arrhythmias.

Dressler's syndrome: an autoimmune pericarditis that has a usual onset of 4–6 weeks post-MI.

SPREAD:

S — Sudden death, shock – hypovolaemia/cardiogenic shock
P — Pericarditis
R — Rupture of papillary muscle/left ventricular free wall. May result in ventricular septal defect/mitral regurgitation
E — Embolism (thromboembolism/thrombus)
A — Arrhythmias and left ventricular aneursym*
D — Dressler's syndrome

*One year on, beware of the patient presenting with persistent ST - elevation — they may have developed a left ventricular aneurysm.

7.2.5 *Long-term management*

Patients should be encouraged to stop smoking, undertake regular exercise, and eat a healthy diet. In addition, all patients should be on aspirin, beta-blocker, ACE inhibitor, and statin in the long term unless contra-indicated. See Chapter 4 *Commonly Encountered Patients* for more details.

7.3 Management of NSTEMI and Unstable Angina

The patient can also present with symptoms of cardiac ischaemia.

Symptoms:

- Crushing central chest pain
- Rest pain (non-exertional chest pain)
- Increasing symptoms of angina

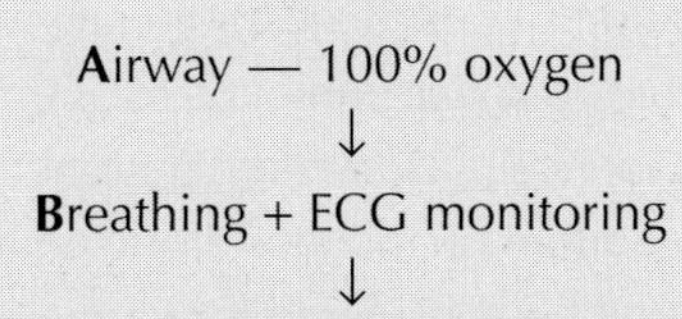

Airway — 100% oxygen

↓

Breathing + ECG monitoring

↓

Circulation (*insert two large bore cannulas into the antecubital fossae and take bloods including FBC, U&Es, troponin, lipids and glucose*)

↓

Give 300 mg aspirin orally and Clopidogrel 300 mg

↓

5–10 mg morphine + 10 mg metoclopramide

↓

2 puffs GTN

↓

Beta-blocker if not contra-indicated (that is, in asthma)

↓

Low molecular weight heparin (LMWH) (for example, enoxaparin 1 mg/kg/12-hourly — twice a day)

Diagnosis depends upon clinical history, serial ECG changes, and biochemical markers of myocardial injury.

Note! Unstable angina can occur in the absence of ECG **and** troponin rise!

Patients with NSTEMI/unstable angina should be risk stratified depending on several factors including their history, clinical examination findings, ECG changes and troponin level. High risk patients should be considered for PCI+/− treatment with a glycoprotein infusion, for example, tirofiban.

Following a STEMI/NSTEMI, **NICE guidelines** recommend that aspirin and clopidogrel be continued for a further 12 months.

All patients should be considered for therapy with aspirin, statin, angiotensin converting enzyme inhibitor (ACEI), and beta-blocker, and patients with evidence of LV systolic dysfunction should also be considered for the addition of an aldosterone antagonist.

All patients should be considered for cardiac revascularisation.

There is good evidence that cardiac rehabilitation is beneficial to patients post-MI and should be available to these patients.

7.4 Management of Arrhythmias

The five-step Immediate Management Plan:

Step 1: Assess **haemodynamic status** — blood pressure, signs of heart failure, urine output, and level of consciousness.
Step 2: Print the **ECG** — you must try to capture the rhythm.
Step 3: Large bore **intravenous access** (very important!).
Step 4: Look for **cause**:

- Send blood including electrolytes — potassium, magnesium and calcium levels.
- Review the drug chart for causative agents.

Step 5: Ensure that the **crash trolley** is nearby!

It is useful to classify the arrhythmia using the rate and QRS complex — see the *Arrhythmias* section of Chapter 4 *Commonly Encountered Patients*.

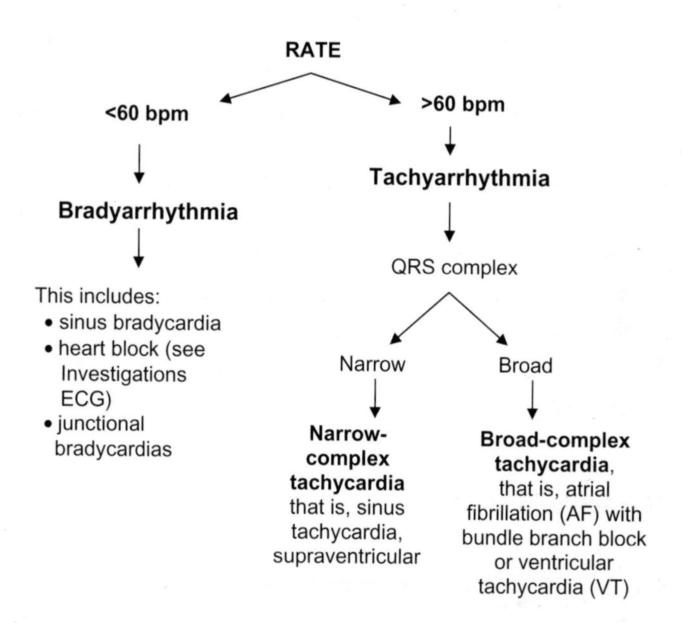

Figure 7.4 Classification of arrhythmias

7.5 Management of Bradyarrhythmias

Bradyarrhythmias include: sinus bradycardia, sinus node disease/ sick sinus node (failure of the sinus node), heart block and junctional bradycardia (AV node acts as pacemaker when sinus node fails).

ECG

If the patient is haemodynamically unstable — give **atropine 1 mg intravenously**.

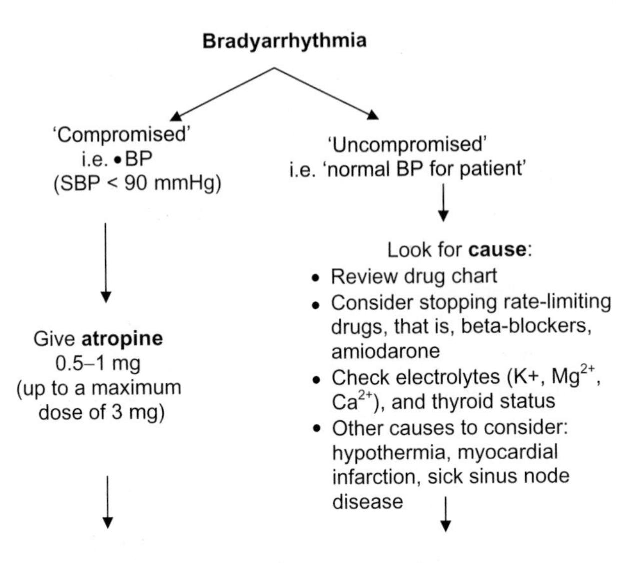

Figure 7.5 Bradyarrhythmias

Consider **pacing**:

- external pacing with defibrillator pads
- temporary pacing wire
- permanent pacing

For more details on pacing — see the 'Pacing' section.

If pacing is delayed, consider starting **Isoprenaline infusion**. **Urgent pacing** is indicated in patients with asystole, or symptomatic bradycardia.

7.6 Management of Tachyarrhythmias

If the patient is haemodynamically unstable then cardiovert — (**D**irect **C**urrent cardioversion) under sedation or general anaesthesia.

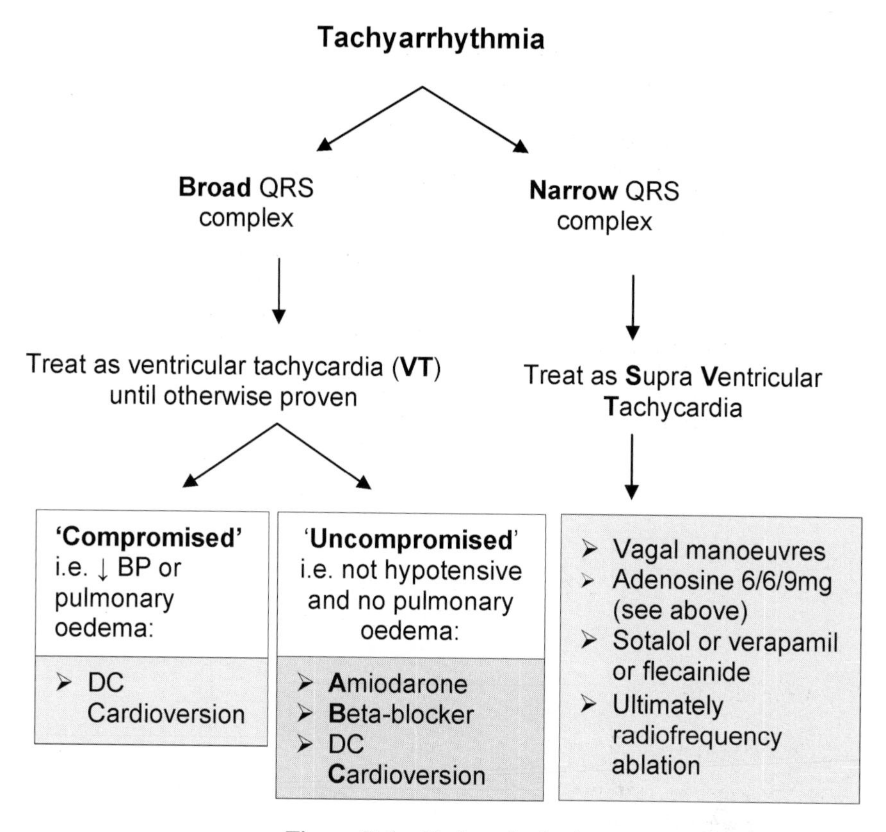

Figure 7.6 Tachyarrhythmias

- **Lignocaine** — may be used to treat ventricular tachycardia (in the absence of severe LV dysfunction) — discuss with senior. It is relatively short acting.
- **Intravenous** bolus of **magnesium** (4–8 mmol) may also help.
- If possible avoid IV **digoxin** and verapamil if Wolff-Parkinson-White syndrome (WPW) suspected.

Chapter 8

Appendix

8.1 ECG Examples

The following pages contain examples of common electrocardiogram (ECG) findings for you to practice with. Begin by covering up the answers at the bottom of the page and work through each ECG systematically as described in chapter 3-*Investigations.*

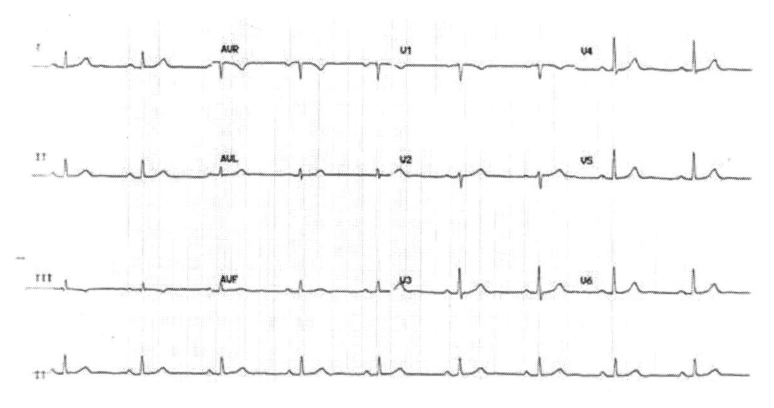

Figure 8.1 What does this ECG show?

Answer: 'Normal' ECG.

Note:

- Familiarise yourself with the features of a normal ECG.
- Practise by going through the ten principles outlined in the *ECG* section of Chapter 3 *Investigations.*
- Note the regularity of the rhythm strips — see lead II.

- Isolated T wave inversions may be seen in leads III, aVR, and VI.
- When confident, move on to the following pages.

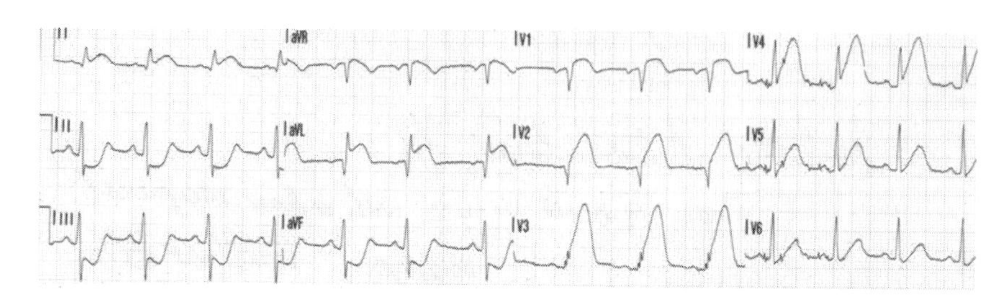

Figure 8.2 What does this ECG show?

Answer: Acute anterior ST-elevation myocardial infarction.

Note:

- ST elevation in the anterior leads (V1–V6).
- Accompanied by reciprocal ST depression in the inferior leads II, III and aVF.
- Likely artery affected: Left anterior descending (LAD).

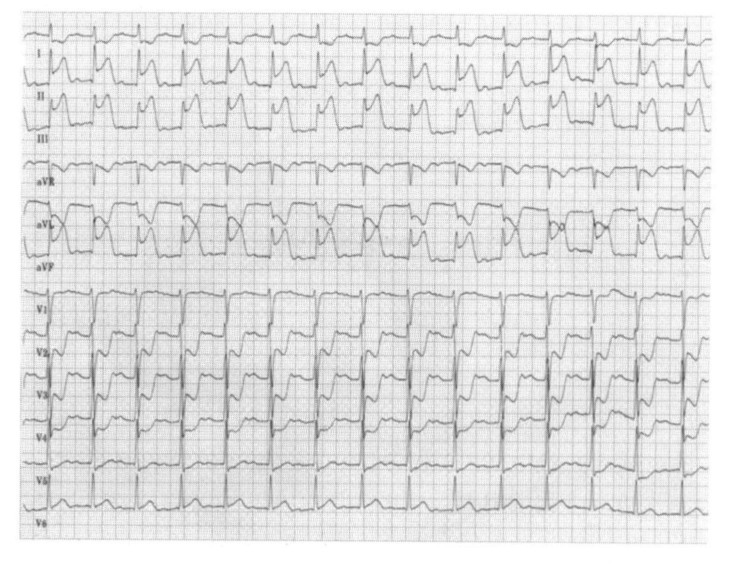

Figure 8.3 What does this ECG show?

Answer: Acute inferior ST-elevation myocardial infarction.

Note:

- ST-elevation in the inferior leads (II, III, and aVF).
- Associated with reciprocal ST-depression — I, aVL and V5.
- Look out for: bradycardia and or heart block.

The affected artery (commonly the right coronary artery — RCA) also supplies the sinoatrial (SA) node thus an inferior infarct can impair the blood supply to the SA node resulting in the conduction defects noted above. Heart block or bradycardia associated with an inferior infarct generally resolves within weeks. Pacing is often not required unless the patient is haemodynamically unstable (that is, low blood pressure, pulmonary oedema). The definitive treatment is restoration of perfusion to the infarcted area, that is, via primary coronary intervention — angioplasty or thrombolysis.

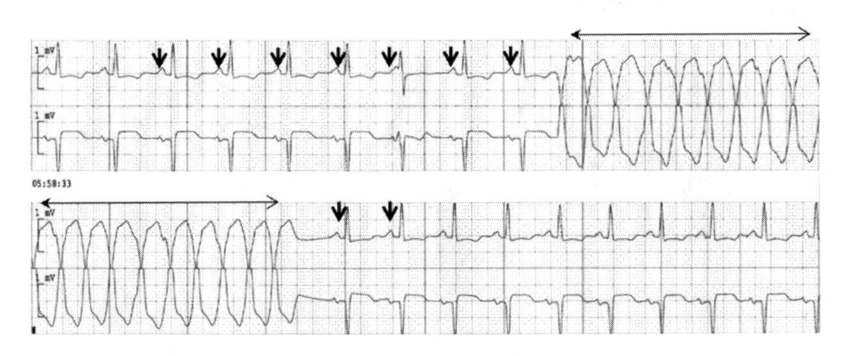

Figure 8.4 What does this ECG show?

Answer: Sinus rhythm degenerates into ventricular tachycardia (VT) with spontaneous returns to sinus rhythm.

Note:

- Short arrows indicate P waves preceding QRS complexes confirming sinus rhythm.
- Long bar indicates beats of broad complex tachycardia — Ventricular Tachycardia (VT).

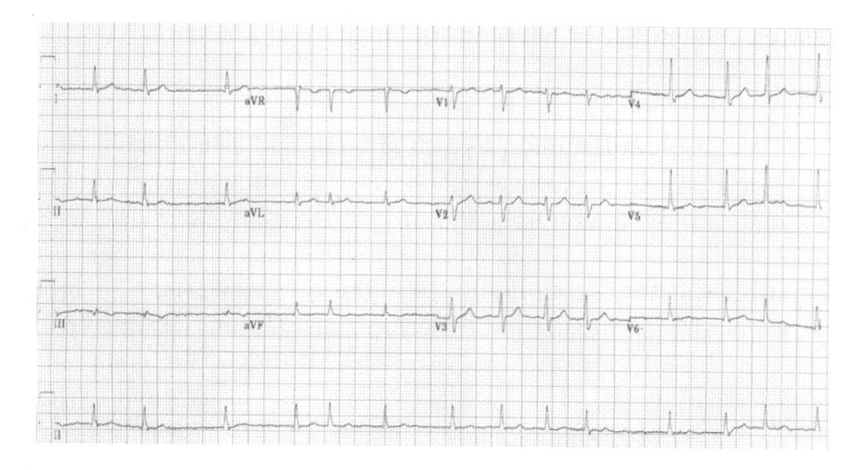

Figure 8.5 What does this ECG show?

Answer: Atrial fibrillation.

Note:

- Irregular ECG — irregular rate.
- No discrete (absent) P waves.
- Broad, irregular QRS complexes (irregular in frequency, size and shape, that is, compare the QRS complex in lead III to lead II).

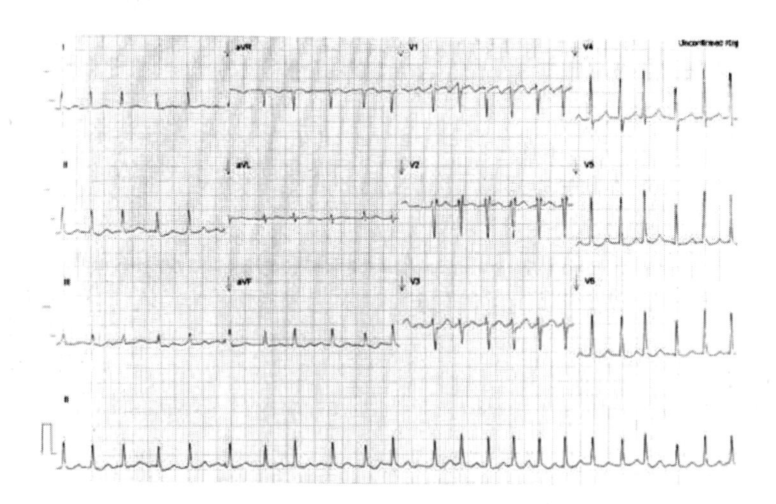

Figure 8.6 What does this ECG show?

Answer: Fast atrial fibrillation.

Note:

- Note the irregularity of this ECG.
- No discrete (absent) P waves.
- Irregular QRS complexes (irregular in frequency, size and shape).
- Always assess the patient — ABC, is the patient haemodynamically stable — refer to chapter 4-*Atrial fibrillation* for patient evaluation.

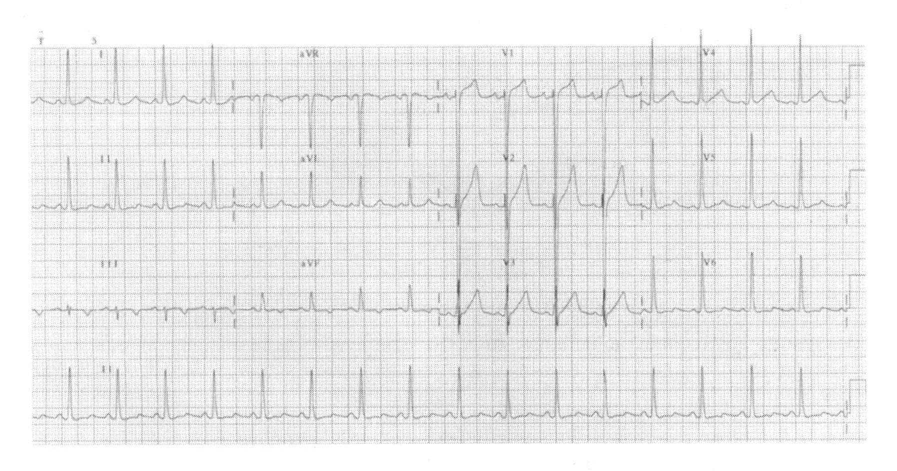

Figure 8.7 What does this ECG show?

Answer: Left ventricular hypertrophy (LVH).

Note:

- Note the tall R waves in the left ventricular leads (see V5 and V6) and deep S waves in the right ventricular leads (see V1 and V2).
- Voltage Criteria $\mathbf{SV_1 + RV_6 > 35\ mm}$ (deep S wave in V1 added to tall R wave in V5/V6 is >7 large squares).

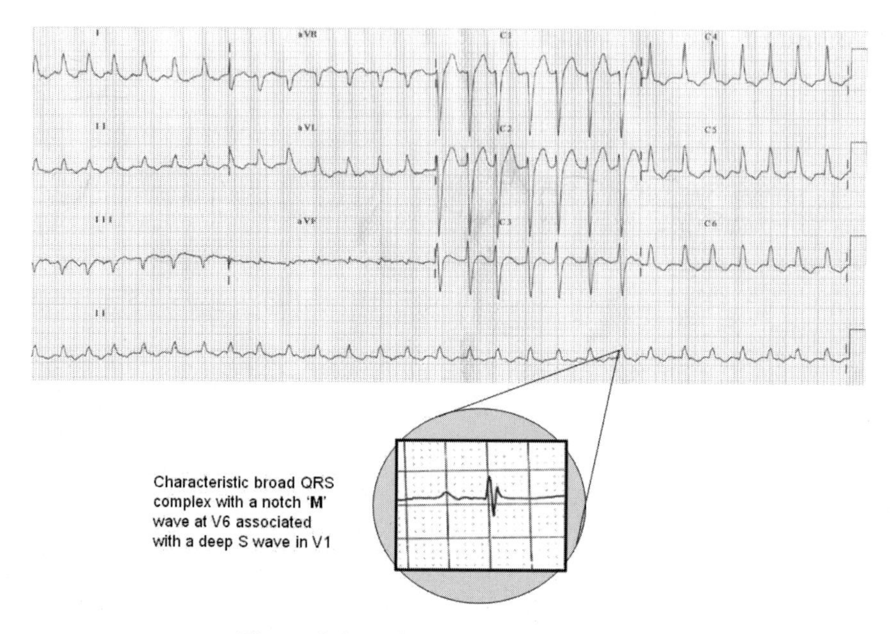

Figure 8.8 What does this ECG show?

Answer: Left bundle branch block (LBBB).

Note:

- Wide 'broad' QRS complexes in all leads.
- '**M**' type QRS complex best seen in leads V5–V6.
- Associated with a deep S wave in lead V1 +/− anterolateral T wave inversion.

If you suspect LBBB on ECG then it is important to determine whether this is '**new**' **LBBB or** '**old**', that is, as is evident from the patient's previous ECGs. Reperfusion (either via percutaneous coronary intervention — angioplasty, or thrombolysis) is indicated in patient presenting with **ischaemic-type chest pain accompanied by 'new' LBBB on ECG**.

Note: Also shows **Left ventricular hypertrophy (LVH)** — see Figure 8.7.

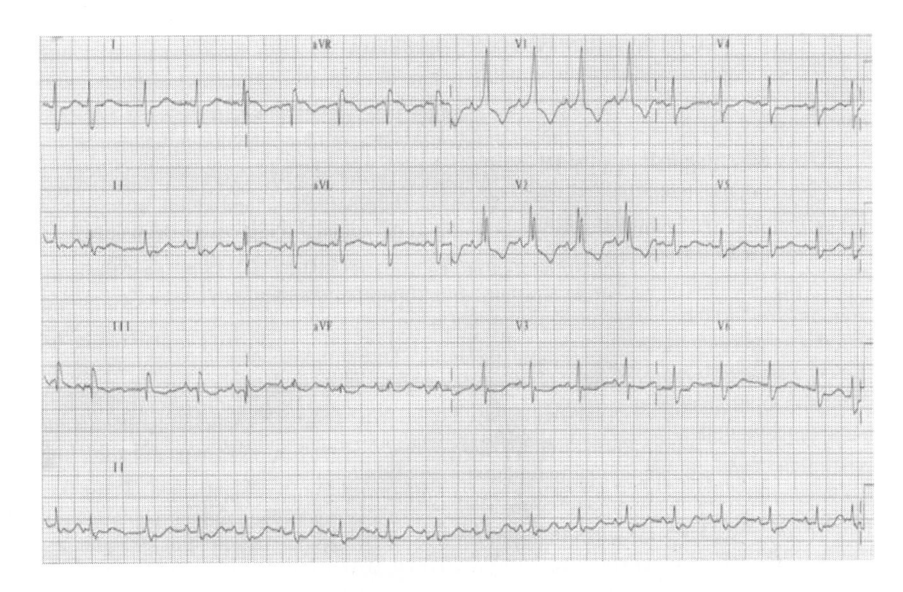

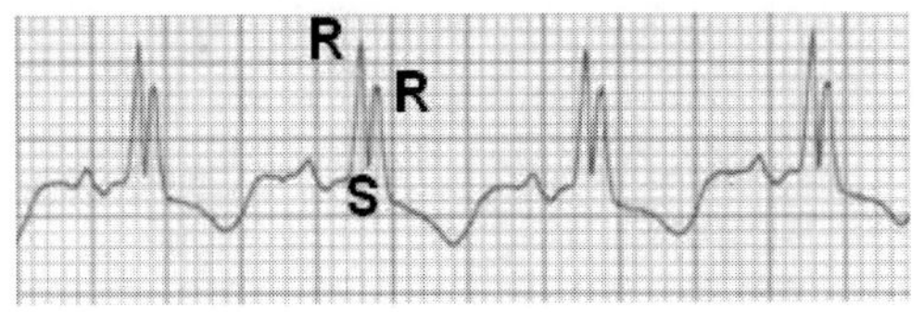

Figure 8.9 What does this ECG show?

Answer: Right bundle branch block (RBBB).

Note:

- Wide 'broad' QRS complexes in all leads.
- An 'M-pattern' is seen in V1 (known formally as an '**RSR**' wave) with a 'W-pattern' in V6 (with a prominent 's' wave).

8.2 How to Measure Blood Pressure

How to measure blood pressure:

- Use an appropriate cuff size (the bladder should encircle at least 80% of the arm but not more than 100%) in order to avoid over- or under-estimation of the blood pressure).
- Palpate the brachial artery and wrap the cuff carefully above the elbow.
- Inflate the cuff until the heart sound disappears completely then deflate the cuff lowering the mercury column slowly (2 mmHg per second) until the heart beat re-appears. This is **Korotkoff phase I — the systolic BP**.
- Continue to deflate by 2 mmHg until the sound becomes muffled and then disappears completely — the complete disappearance of the heart sound is **Korotkoff phase V, the Diastolic BP**. Round-off your measurement to the nearest 2 mmHg, that is, 126/84 mmHg.

8.3 Some Important Principles in Cardiology

Cardiac output is the amount of blood ejected from the heart usually measured in litres per minute. The amount of blood that is ejected by the left ventricle following one contraction is known as the stroke volume. Therefore, the following relationship holds:

$$\mathbf{CO = SV \times HR}$$

where:

CO = cardiac output in L/min
SV = stroke volume per beat
HR = heart rate

$$\mathbf{MAP = (CO \times SVR) + CVP}$$

where:

MAP = mean arterial pressure
SVR = systemic vascular resistance
CVP = central venous pressure

At rest, the MAP can be approximated by measuring the systolic and diastolic pressures.

$$\mathbf{MAP = DP + 1/3(SP - DP)}$$

where:

DP = diastolic pressure
SP = systolic pressure

The MAP is generally regarded as the perfusion pressure and a value above 60 mmHg is necessary for sufficient perfusion to the organs.

The Frank-Starling's law is probably one of the most important principles in cardiology you should familiarise yourself with. It is useful to be able to reproduce the simple graph below.

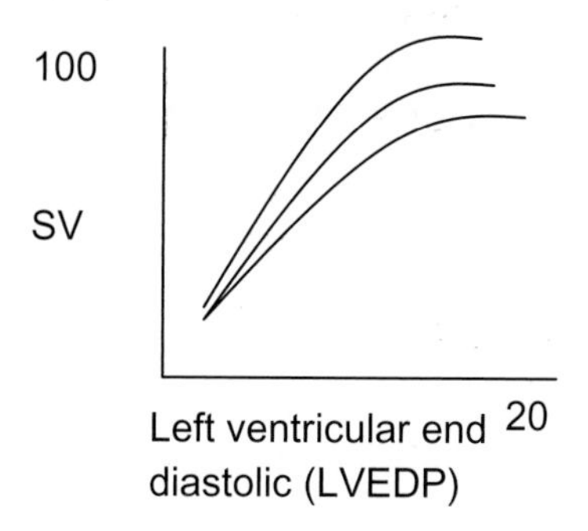

The law states that the greater the volume of blood entering the heart during diastole, that is, the **end diastolic volume**, the greater the volume of blood ejected during systolic contraction, otherwise known as the **stroke volume**. This is because the end diastolic volume is determined by the **preload**, which refers to the tension of the myocyte fibres *prior* to contraction. (Note: **Afterload** refers to the tension required for the ventricle to contract.) The more the fibres are stretched, the greater the sarcomere length and the bigger the force of contraction. But as you can see from the graph, this proportional relationship only exists up to a certain point beyond which the myocytes can no longer accommodate the increase in end diastolic volume.

8.4 Brugada Syndrome

This is characterised by:

- right bundle branch block (see Fig. 8.9)
- ST segment elevation in V1 to V3
- +/− syncope or sudden death

8.5 Dietary Approaches to Stop Hypertension (DASH)

The **DASH** diet is an example of a non-pharmacological anti-hypertensive lifestyle modification. Sacks *et al.* showed that reduction in dietary salt (sodium) intake, alongside measures such as: eating more fruits and vegetables, reducing saturated fat and total fat intake and eating less red meat resulted in a reduction in blood pressure.

8.6 Jervell and Lange-Nielsen Syndrome

This is a congenital cause of prolonged QT interval (long QT syndrome). It is *autosomal recessively inherited* and is associated with syncope/sudden death and congenital deafness.

8.7 Romano-Ward Syndrome

This is another congenital cause of prolonged QT interval (long QT syndrome). It is *autosomal dominantly inherited* and is associated with syncope or sudden death.

References

Antithrombotic Trialists' Collaboration. Collaborative meta-analysis of randomised trials of antiplatelet therapy for prevention of death, myocardial infarction, and stroke in high risk patients. *Br Med J* 2002 Jan 12;324(7329):71–86. Erratum in: *Br Med J* 2002 Jan 19; 324(7330):141.

Brady A.J., Betteridge D.J. Prevalence and risks of undertreatment with statins. *Br J Cardiol* 2003;10(3):218–9.

British Hypertension Society. www.bhsoc.org (last accessed 18 May 2009).

British Hypertension Society. http://www.bhsoc.org/Cardiovascular_Risk_Prediction_Chart.stm (last accessed 25 May 2009).

Camm J.A., *et al.* Prevention of Cardiovascular Disease European Society of Cardiology, Oxford, 2007.

CAPRIE Steering Committee. A randomised, blinded, trial of clopidogrel versus aspirin in patients at risk of ischaemic events. *Lancet* 1997 Nov 16;348(9038):1329–39.

Chilson D., Cannom D.S., Moore R. Design and results of the Antiarrhythmics vs. Implantable Defibrillators (AVID) Registry. *Circulation* 1999;99: 1692–1699.

Cohn J.N., Tognoni G. Valsartan Heart Failure Trial Investigators. A randomised trial of the angiotensin-receptor blocker valsartan in chronic heart failure. *N Engl J Med* 2001 Dec 6;345(23):1667–75.

Connolly S., Gent M., Roberts R. For the CIDS investigators. Canadian Implantable Defibrillator Study (CIDS). A randomised trial of the implantable cardioverter defibrillator against amiodarone. *Circulation* 2000;101:1297–1302.

Dahlöf B., Sever P.S., Poulter N.R., Wedel H., *et al.* For the ASCOT investigators. Prevention of cardiovascular events with an antihypertensive regimen of amlodipine adding perindopril as required versus atenolol adding bendroflumethiazide as required, in the Anglo-Scandinavian Cardiac Outcomes Trial-Blood Pressure Lowering Arm (ASCOT-BPLA): a multicentre randomised controlled trial. *Lancet* 2005;366: 895–906.

Dargie H.J. Effect of carvedilol on outcome after myocardial infarction in patients with left-ventricular dysfunction: the CAPRICORN randomised trial. *Lancet* 2001 May 5;357(9266):1385–90.

Dargie H.J., Ford I., Fox K.M. Total Ischaemic Burden European Trial (TIBET). Effects of ischaemia and treatment with atenolol, nifedipine SR and their combination on outcome in patients with chronic stable angina. The TIBET Study Group. *Eur Heart J* 1996 Jan;17(1): 104–12.

Doshi R.N., Daoud E.G., Fellows C., Turk K., Duran A., Hamdan M.H., Pires L.A. PAVE Study Group. Left ventricular-based cardiac stimulation post AV nodal ablation evaluation (the PAVE study). *J Cardiovasc Electrophysiol* 2005 Nov;16(11):1160–5.

Drake R., Vogl A., Mitchell A., *et al.* (2008). *Gray's Atlas of Anatomy*, Churchill Livingstone, Philadelphia.

Eichhorn E.J., Bristow M.R. The Carvedilol Prospective Randomised Cumulative Survival (COPERNICUS) trial. *Curr Control Trials Cardiovasc Med* 2001;2(1):20–23.

El-Chami M.F., Grow P., Eilen D., Lerakis S., Block P.C. Clinical outcomes three years after PLAATO implantation. *Catheter Cardiovasc Interv* 2007 Apr 1;69(5):704–7.

Fibrinolytic Therapy Trialists' (FTT) Collaborative Group Indications for fibrinolytic therapy in suspected acute myocardial infarction: collaborative overview of early mortality and major morbidity results from all randomised trials of more than 1000 patients. *Lancet* 1994 Feb 5;343(8893):311–22.

Final report on the aspirin component of the ongoing Physicians' Health Study. Steering Committee of the Physicians' Health Study Research Group. *N Engl J Med* 1989 Jul 20;321(3):129–35. *Br Med J* 2002 12 Jan;324:71–86.

Hall S.A., Cigarroa C.G., Marcoux L., Risser R.C., *et al.* Time course of improvement in left ventricular function, mass and geometry in patients with congestive heart failure treated with beta-adrenergic blockade. *J Am Coll Cardiol* 1995;25(5):1154–61.

Hampton J.R. (2003). *ECG Made Easy*, Churchill Livingstone.

Hjalmarson A., Goldstein S., Fagerberg B., Wedel H., Waagstein F., Kjekshus J., Wikstrand J., El Allaf D., Vítovec J., Aldershvile J., Halinen M., Dietz R., Neuhaus K.L., Jánosi A., Thorgeirsson G., Dunselman P.H., Gullestad L., Kuch J., Herlitz J., Rickenbacher P., Ball S,, Gottlieb S., Deedwania P. Effects of controlled-release metoprolol on total mortality, hospitalizations, and well-being in patients with heart failure: the Metoprolol CR/XL Randomised Intervention Trial in congestive heart failure (MERIT-HF). MERIT-HF Study Group. *J Am Med Assoc* 2000 Mar 8;283(10):1295–302.

ISIS-2. 10 year survival among patients with suspected acute myocardial infarction in randomised comparison of intravenous streptokinase, oral aspirin, both, or neither. *Br Med J* 1998 2 May;316:1337–43.

ISIS-2 (Second International Study of Infarct Survival) Collaborative Group. Randomised trial of intravenous streptokinase, oral aspirin, both, or neither among 17,187 cases of suspected acute myocardial infarction: ISIS-2. *Lancet* 1988 Aug 13;2(8607):349–60.

ISIS-4. A randomised factorial trial assessing early oral captopril, oral mononitrate, and intravenous magnesium sulphate in 58,050 patients with suspected acute myocardial infarction. ISIS-4 (Fourth International Study of Infarct Survival) Collaborative Group. *Lancet* 1995 Mar 18; 345(8951):669–85.

Joint Working Group on Coronary Angioplasty of the British Cardiac Society and British Cardiovascular Intervention Society. Coronary angioplasty: guidelines for good practice and training. *Heart* 2007;83: 224–35.

Moore K., Agur A. (1995). *Essential Clinical Anatomy*, Lippincott Williams & Wilkins, Baltimore.

Moss A.J., Hall W.J., Cannom D.S., Daubert J.P., Higgins S.L., Klein H., Levine J.H., Saksena S., Waldo A.L., Wilber D., Brown M.W., Heo M. Improved survival with an implanted defibrillator in patients with coronary disease at high risk for ventricular arrhythmia. Multicenter automatic defibrillator implantation trial investigators. *N Engl J Med* 1996 Dec 26;335(26):1933–40.

Nashef S.A.M., Rogues F., Michel P., Gauducheau E., *et al.* European system for cardiac operative risk evaluation (EuroSCORE). *Eur J Cardiothorac Surg* 1999;16:9–13.

National Institute for Health Clinical Excellence. www.nice.org.uk (last accessed 18 May 2009).

Newby D.E. (2005). *Cardiology: An Illustrated Colour Text*, Elsevier.

Nolan J., *et al.* (2008). *Advanced Life Support*, 5th Edn., Resuscitation Council, London.

Opie L.H. (2005). *Drugs for the Heart*, 6th Edn., Resuscitation Council, London.

Packer M., Gheorghiade M., Young J.B., Costantini P.J., Adams K.F., Cody R.J., Smith L.K., Van Voorhees L., Gourley L.A., Jolly M.K. Withdrawal of digoxin from patients with chronic heart failure treated with angiotensin-converting-enzyme inhibitors. RADIANCE Study. *N Engl J Med* 2003 Jul 1;329(1):1–7.

Pepine C.J., Handberg-Thurmond E., Marks R.G., Conlon M., Cooper-DeHoff R., Volkers P., Zellig P. (1998). Rationale and design of the International Verapamil SR/Trandolapril Study (INVEST): an Internet-based randomized trial in coronary artery disease patients with hypertension. *J Am Coll Cardiol* Nov;32(5):1228–37.

Pitt B., Zannad F., Remme W.J., Cody R., *et al.* The effect of apironolactone on morbidity and mortality in patients with severe heart failure. Radomized Aldactone Evaluation Study Investigators. *N Engl J Med* 1999;341(10):709–17.

Pitt B., Segal R., Martinez F., Meurers G., Cowley A., Thomas I., Deedwania P., *et al.* Randomised trial of losartan versus captopril in patients over 65 with heart failure (Evaluation of Losartan in the Elderly Study, ELITE). *Lancet* 1997;349(9054):747–52.

Ramrakha P., Moore K. (2004). *Oxford Handbook of Acute Medicine*, 2nd Edn., Oxford University Press, Oxford.

Ramrakha P. (2007). *Oxford Handbook of Cardiology*, Oxford University Press.

Rehnqvist N., Hjemdahl P., Billing E., Björkander I., Eriksson S.V., Forslund L., Held C., Näsman P., Wallén N.H. Effects of metoprolol vs verapamil in patients with stable angina pectoris. The Angina Prognosis

Study in Stockholm (APSIS). *Eur Heart J* 1996 Jan;17(1):76–81. Erratum in: *Eur Heart J* 1996 Mar;17(3):483.

Rovelli F., De Vita C., Feruglio G.A., Lotto A., Selvini A., Tognoni G. GISSI trial: early results and late follow-up. Gruppo Italiano per la Sperimentazione della Streptochinasi nell'Infarto Miocardico. *J Am Coll Cardiol* 1987 Nov;10(5 Suppl B):33B–39B.

Sacks F.M., Pfeffer M.A., Moye L.A., Rouleau J.L., Rutherford J.D., Cole T.G., Brown L.,Warnica J.W., Arnold J.M., Wun C.C., Davis B.R., Braunwald E. The effect of pravastatin on coronary events after myocardial infarction in patients with average cholesterol levels. Cholesterol and Recurrent Events Trial investigators. *N Engl J Med* 1996 Oct 3;335(14):1001–9.

Scottish Intercollegiate Guidelines Network (SIGN). Cardiac arrhythmias in coronary heart disease. A national clinical guideline. Edinburgh, 2007.

Sever P.S., Dahlöf B., Poulter N.R. *et al.* Prevention of coronary and stroke events with atorvastatin in hypertensive patients who have average or lower-than-average cholesterol concentrations, in the Anglo-Scandinavian Cardiac Outcomes Trial-Lipid Lowering Arm (ASCOT-LLA): a multicentre randomised controlled trial. *Lancet* 2003 Apr 5;361(9364):1149–58.

Swanton R.H. (2003). *Cardiology Pocket Consultant*, Wiley-Blackwell.

The ALLHAT Officers and Coordinators for the ALLHAT Collaborative Research Group. Major outcomes in high-risk hypertensive patients randomised to angiotensin converting enzyme inhibitor or calcium channel blocker vs diuretic. *Journal of the American Medical Association* 2002;288:2981–97.

The Antiarrhythmics versus Implantable Defibrillators (AVID) Investigators. A comparison of antiarrhythmic-drug therapy with implantable defibrillators in patients resuscitated from near-fatal ventricular arrhythmias. *N Engl J Med* 1997 Nov 27;337(22):1576–83.

The Cardiac Insufficiency Bisoprolol Study II (CIBIS-II). A randomised trial. *Lancet* 1999 Jan 2;353(9146):9–13.

The CONSENSUS Trial Study Group. Effects of enalapril on mortality in severe congestive heart failure. Results of the Cooperative North

Scandinavian Enalapril Survival Study (CONSENSUS). *N Engl J Med* 1987 Jun 4;316(23):1429–35.

The Scandinavian Simvastatin Survival Study. Randomised trial of cholesterol lowering in 4444 patients with coronary heart disease. *Lancet* 1994 Nov 19;344(8934):1383–9.

Wilhelmsen L., Berglund G., Elmfeldt D., *et al.* Beta-blockers versus diuretics in hypertensive men: main results from the HAPPHY trial. *Am J Hypertens* 1987;5:561–72.

World Health Organisation. www.who.int (last accessed 18 May 2009).

Wyse D.G., Talajic M., Hafley G.E., Buxton A.E., *et al.* Antiarrhythmic drug therapy in the Multicenter UnSustained Tachycardia Trial (MUSTT): drug testing and as-treated analysis. *J Am Coll Cardiol* 2001;38:344–351.

Yusuf S., Sleight P., Pogue J., Bosch J., Davies R., Dagenais G. Effects of an angiotensin-converting-enzyme inhibitor, ramipril, on cardiovascular events in high-risk patients. The heart outcomes prevention evaluation study investigators. *N Engl J Med* 2000 Jan 20;342(3):145–53.

Index